man on top

lose fat, get fit, and control your weight for life

Roland Denzel, Precision Nutrition-PnC, IKFF-CKT

with

Galina Ivanova Denzel, NSCA-CPT, RES

Disclaimer

You must get your doctor's approval before beginning this diet and exercise program.

This book/ebook provides information that you read and use at your own risk. We do not take responsibility for any misfortune that may happen, either directly or indirectly, from reading and applying the information contained and/or referenced in this book/ebook. The programs and information expressed within this book/ebook are NOT medical advice, but rather represent the authors' opinions, and are solely for informational and educational purposes.

Please do not use the information in this book without first discussing your fitness, training, and nutrition plans with a qualified doctor or health practitioner. The authors are not responsible for any injury or health condition that may occur through following the programs and opinions expressed within this book. The dietary information is presented for informational purposes only and may not be appropriate for all individuals.

Remember; consult with your physician before starting *any* exercise program or altering your diet.

Table of Contents

Dedication

To my moms.

Meredith – who never saw me thin and fit, but tried hard to help me become so. As a type 1 diabetic, my mom lived a healthy lifestyle herself, and gave me a good example to follow. I just refused. Meredith passed away in 2002, while I was still fat, but after I'd lost the first five of my eventual seventy five pounds lost; she was rooting for me!

Gerry – who lead by example all of my life, and continues to do so, today. Gerry is a cancer survivor and reference librarian, who inspires me to do my own nutrition research, make informed decisions, and take health matters into my own hands, rather than take what "they" say as gospel. Always active and fit, a healthy eater and wonderful cook, Gerry couldn't be a better influence or a better mom.

Pepa, Galya's mother – who raised such a wonderful daughter in Galya, instilling in her a sense of purpose and a drive to work hard. Despite the hard times and tough conditions, Pepa was able to raise a happy, warm, and caring woman who loves, helps, and cares for others above all else.

Acknowledgments

The biggest acknowledgment has to go to my wife, Galya Ivanova Denzel, who has influenced me more than I could have ever imagined. I can't imagine a partner (and writing partner) better suited to my own idiosyncrasies. She's smart and pretty, but she's also patient when I'm not and perfectly impatient when I need a kick in the tail.

I cringe at the thought of leaving someone out, so I can't risk starting a list of those who've been there for me, all along my ten year journey from an overweight couch potato to fitness writer, nutrition coach, and trainer. It's just too long.

When it comes to this book, I've had encouragement, inspiration, and plenty of help! Thanks to Lou Schuler, Adam Campbell, Dave Sisler, Dan John, Nick Bromberg, Chris Bathke, Tony Sayers, John Gesselberty, Gabe Wilson, Charlie Shnosky III, "Mighty" Joe Stankowski, Erika Warriner, Steve Cotter, Alan Aragon, John Berardi, Robin Luethe, Jesus, Bill Snell, Tina Kinsley, Jill Janssen, Jane Gsellman, Wendy Welch, Ginger Eichstadt, Kevin Larabee, Ryan Oddo, Hal Johnson, Michael and Jamie Wilson, and Bill Hartman. Special thanks to Peter Lutes for his eagle-eyed reading, Sean Hendrickson for his great and patient website work, and to Eugene Bachelder for being my training partner in front of the camera. Finally, to Jean-Paul Francoeur, who consistently and repeatedly asked me *when* I was going to write a book, and never *if*.

– Roland

This book would have only been an idea without all the help, support, faith and encouragement we got along the way.

I would like to thank my husband and partner in culinary crime Roland Denzel, who is fun, supportive and always knows how to translate what I say in a way that men will understand. In my growth as a coach I am forever grateful to Bill Hartman, who taught me much about quality of movement and personal dedication, Katy Bowman, who's been an extraordinary influence in my view of natural movement, and all my clients who worked hard and allowed me to learn with them and through them.

Thanks to Lou Schuler, who kept us real and believed in us. More thanks to Alan Aragon, John Berardi, Alwyn Cosgrove, Adam Campbell, Chris Bathke, JP Francoeur, Diana Shingarova, Dinko Stranski, Steve Cotter, Eftim Iliev, Gergana Paraskova, Spas Smilenov.

– Galya

Foreword – by Lou Schuler

Roland Denzel is one of my heroes. His transformation from overweight and sedentary to muscular and active is impressive in itself, but that's only part of the story.

I first met Roland at The Fitness Summit in 2006 in Little Rock, Arkansas. On the last day of the Summit our host, Jean-Paul Francoeur, led us on a hike to a small hilltop overlooking the Arkansas River. Roland and I were somewhere in the middle of the pack, and had a long conversation about ... something. I just remember thinking Roland was a good guy at the front end of a personal journey of some sort. He used to be one thing, and he wanted to be something else, and he was closer to the first than the second.

We stayed in touch via email, mostly talking about family-guy things, and met again at the 2008 Summit. For me, the Summit was one of a series of fun and successful events. I'd been to every one since 2004, and I took away useful information and good memories from each. But for Roland, it was epic. He met Galya, his future wife, and he got hooked on training with kettlebells, thanks to Steve Cotter, the featured presenter.

Roland got certified as a kettlebell instructor through Steve's organization, and courted Galya in earnest. I don't know if the two pursuits—love and exercise—were separate tracks on his personal journey, or if they were somehow part of the same path. Whatever happened, it transformed him from a nice guy working to get in shape to a genuine fitness pro who looks and lives the part.

Without really thinking about it, I found myself asking Roland to preview early drafts of my book chapters, and relying more and more on his knowledge of fitness and nutrition. More than once he led me to key sources of information that I used for magazine articles. And when he did a presentation on kettlebell training at the 2011 Fitness Summit in Kansas City, I never stopped to think how remarkable it was that the guy who still seemed lost in 2006 was now helping others find their way.

That's why I consider Roland not just a success story, but a genuine role model for the many, many men who've allowed themselves to get soft in middle age. It's one thing to succeed at an endeavor and then go off to enjoy your hard-earned and richly deserved success—to live happily ever after, as the stories go. It's something else altogether to dedicate yourself to helping others achieve the same thing.

I hope you enjoy Man on Top. But most of all I hope you see the true message of Roland's story: What he accomplished is entire possible for almost all of you. The only reason it's an anomaly is because it's so rare. Why is it rare? Probably because it's hard, especially when most of the people who write about fitness and nutrition have never actually been in your position. They tend to be people like me, who got into exercise and healthy living at a young age and have never strayed far from the path we chose. It's a great path for accumulating a lot of information and expertise, but knowing things isn't the same as experiencing things.

Roland has that experience. He's been where you are. He's now where I am. There's no one I know who's in a better position to help you get from where you are to where you want to be.

That's why he's one of my heroes.

Lou Schuler, June 2, 2012

Introduction

What was my inspiration to write this book? The 30,000 foot answer is that I feel like I can help you. If you're reading this, it's very likely that you're overweight and out of shape. Well, that was me for most of my life. I've been there, lived there, and finally got out of there, just a few years ago. I'd never been a man on top of anything.

My journey out of "there" began in earnest about 10 years ago, and while I have done a lot of looking back, for the most part it was to take note of how I did it and to wonder why I hadn't done it earlier. For the first time in my life, I feel "on top." Why did I wait so long?

Man on top

Yeah, don't think I'm something I'm not, or worse, don't think that *I think* I'm something I'm not. I'm not really the alpha male type, so I'm not on top like *that*. I'm not a business leader, infomercial salesman, or cult leader, either. I'm not even the type of husband to proclaim "I'm in charge!" (although I am when she lets me). No, my version of being on top is being *on top of things*; taking charge of my own life and health as high level goals, down to the specifics on exercise and diet to support those goals.

This book is to inspire you, the reader, to get lean, slim, ripped, jacked, buff, tight, huge, or even (if it's your thing) healthy. It's to teach you a thing or two about yourself, while keeping you sane, happy, and healthy – all the while, keeping your family and friends sane and happy. That way, they'll be happy for you and all will be right with the world.

This book was written to build or rebuild confidence, as only a man confident in his abilities to change will enact lasting change. This book is to put you on top, whether it's on top *again*, or on top for the first time.

Me

I was fat for most of my adult life and chubby for most of my childhood. There were some short periods where I wasn't fat, but those were few and far between.

When I talk about my fat days, many of my friends tell me that I wasn't really all that fat, but pictures tell a different story.

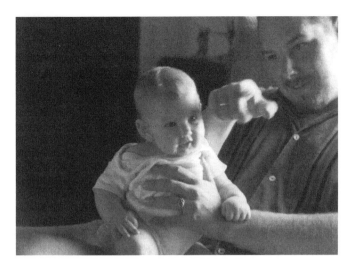

Hey, maybe they were just being nice? Maybe it's that I wasn't fat by comparison to modern day man, so I looked pretty "okay." Who knows?

I was also a pretty down and sad kid. I used to think that getting slim would make me happy. I'm sure I'm not the only one like this, but I would constantly daydream about being "normal," and how happy I would be once I *was* normal. It wasn't until years later that I realized that it was the reverse that was true, and that happiness could lead to being slim. I'll bet that for many overweight people, the subconscious realization that they won't automatically end up happy at the end of their diet does a little something to their motivation to continue. Battling hunger takes willpower based on reality, and down deep we know that the lack of abs isn't keeping us sad.

Then there's getting the girl. I'm sure I'm not the only guy who was overweight and knew that the extra weight was the "only thing" standing between him and a relationship with *that* girl. If not getting the girl doesn't make you sad, then what does? It's a vicious circle of feeling like you never had a chance, followed by anger, sadness, ice cream, wallowing in self-pity, and the inevitable weight gain, after which you're bound to find another girl that you can't have, so just hit "repeat."

The health and nutrition community writes, talks, reports, and blogs about metabolic syndrome, and how it's a vicious circle of insulin resistance, fat gain, slowing metabolism, etc. But, I think the real vicious circle is in our heads – the heads of the overweight. Which comes first, the weight, the sadness, or no girl? Once fat, you get sadder and sadder, fatter and fatter, and despite your mom telling you that "you're very handsome, and any girl would be lucky to have you," being fat is a big barrier between you and that girl.

I got older, slimmer, fatter, older, slightly slimmer, fatter, older and fatter still. I went through lots of ups and downs over the years, and I can now see a correlation between my happier times and my weight. I did get married, and I have two wonderful kids – kids who play a big part in my final desire to finally get the weight off for good.

One day my daughter asked for a glass of water, so I went down to get it, came back up the stairs and sat down. I guess I was huffing and puffing, because my daughter said "you didn't have to run!" I hadn't, I'd merely gone up a few stairs, and ended up pretty winded.

I didn't go on a diet that next day, but it did start me thinking about things. Was I setting a good example? Would my kids end up fat? Would my kids be unhappy? Would they end up lonely like I was? I didn't even think about whether I would be around for them until later, but when my Mom was diagnosed with cancer soon after, everything hit home hard. I took longer and longer looks at where I was, how I felt, and how I looked, and finally decided to do something about it.

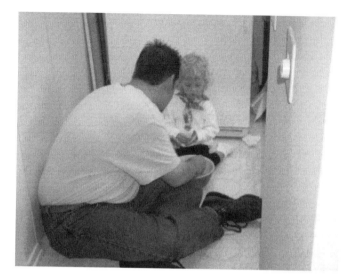

You

I'm not so cocky as to think that I know you. I barely know me. But, if you're reading this book, I'd like to think that we have some things in common, even if we've led totally different lives. I was a sedentary, computer playing, Dungeons & Dragons kid, while you might have been an athlete. I'm a husband and a dad of two and you might be just out of school, recently married, a new empty nester, or even a grandfather.

We are each our own person, but we have something in common – we have weight to lose. We want to get in shape. Many of us have been in shape before, and lost it. For some this will be the first time actually getting fit.

Yeah, I don't know each of you, but I know enough about "us" to help you like I helped myself. I know how I lost the weight, and kept it off. Over the years, many people have asked me how I did it, and how they can do it too. I've found that I almost never tell them what to do. Instead, I often say "Well, what I did was _____." I share the whats and the hows, but most importantly, the whys. If you know why something works, why it doesn't, why it's important, why it's trivial, why it's important to you, and why it rings true, you're going to do it.

Me, today

Fast forward from 2002, when I was still fat, and I feel like I'm almost a different person; I'm a lot leaner, stronger, happier, and healthier. I lost the weight and kept it off, and I've even gotten to the point where I no longer see myself as fat when I look in the mirror. In fact, until about three years ago, I was still reading magazine tips on how to dress to look more slim, even though I probably needed to read the tips on how to look *less* skinny.

After getting skinny, I decided to get stronger and play around with lifting weights. Over time, and following the keen advice of my now friend Lou Schuler, I went from a skinny-fat 160 pounds to a lean and more muscular 195.

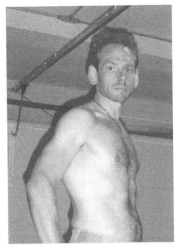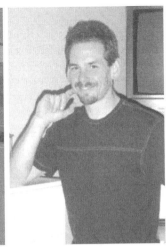

A few years ago, my friends Chris Bathke and Steve Cotter introduced me to kettlebells, encouraging me to use them as part of my training programs. Eventually, I got so interested in kettlebells that I even got certified in how to train with them.

I really love training, which is why I got certified to train people, but I also realized early on that where people *really* need the help is on the eating side of things. People just don't know what the real deal is. ...and it's not our fault; we were simply taught wrong, given false hopes, and bad direction.

During our lifetime, the government's diet and lifestyle recommendations have been based on test tube science and wishful thinking, with no real world experience applied. Just look at the latest recommendation from the USDA, or the United States Department of Agriculture, and their latest slogan – from myplate.org – for slim living and weight loss:

66

"Enjoy Your Food, But Eat Less" – the government

99

This is the USDA's latest advice, just out for 2012, but if memory serves, the past recommendations were *also* to not overeat. If this advice really worked, people wouldn't be overweight, now would they? When I was fat, I tried "but eat less." I'll bet you tried it, too. I'll bet it didn't work any better for you than it did for me.

I know many of us don't really turn directly to the government for our dietary recommendations, but there is a trickle-down effect at work. What they say up high, influences regulations at schools, in hospitals, and even in the military. We learn from this exposure from a young age in school, then as adults via television and entertainment magazine "experts." It's hard to unlearn this stuff!

I believe that these TV doctors really do mean well, but they don't usually do their own research or fact checking, and often get their own nutrition and health information funneled in through advertisers, food companies, and drug manufacturers. They mean well, but some just drop the ball.

Don't get me wrong, true nutrition experts don't discard what the USDA says, just because it's the government. Instead, they take it in, do their own research, and then apply what they learn to real life – real world clients and real world situations – people and pictures vs test tubes and numbers.

Like many frustrated people in this internet day and age, I stopped getting news and further "education" from television and started looking more toward online sources, which contain the convenience of links, references, and email addresses that are merely a click away. I had recently used the internet to become an online friend of Lou's, and soon I was following the *real food* advice of Lou's cowriter and cohort, Adam Campbell.

Adam, now the Fitness Director at Men's Health Magazine, had some stellar dietary advice, which he turned into a great book – Men's Health TNT Diet. Further, Adam's encouragement is what really pushed me over the fitness and nutrition edge, and because of

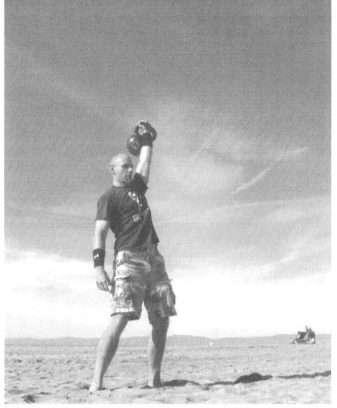

Adam, I decided to be more than just a fitness enthusiast, but to take up nutrition as a profession.

Since Adam's TNT, I feel like I've read , tried, or applied every diet in the bookstore *and* every plan I could find on the internet; I learned from each one, and along the way made friends with many enthusiasts, professionals, and experts in the nutrition world. I learned a lot from them, and even decided to become certified myself, choosing John Berardi's Precision Nutrition Certification (Pn1) because of its focus on positive habit forming.

In ten years, I've seen what works and what doesn't, but more importantly, I've seen what works well, what works more easily, more healthfully, and more efficiently. I've seen what works to get the weight off and then keep it off.

It's been a long time since I was overweight. Today, I have friends that don't know I was *ever* fat, and when they look shocked when I tell them about it, it's a great feeling.

For most of you, this book will not be your first attempt to lose weight. We've lost before, and here we are again.

Let this be the last time; you're going to lose the weight and keep it off. In ten years, drop me a line and tell me that you're still where you want to be.

Why I didn't write this book alone

I've wanted to write this book for a long time. I feel like I have the information that you can use to get slim and fit like I did. I feel like I can explain it in such a way that you can take it in and immediately put it into practice. But, I'm just one guy who lost weight. Just because I did it for me doesn't mean that the same things are going to work for you. So, who am I to write this book?

A few years ago, at a fitness seminar, I met a trainer, writer, nutrition coach, chef, and gym owner from Bulgaria. As she is a Bulgarian trainer and coach, with the exotic Bond-girl sounding name of Galina Ivanova Ivanova (yes, two Ivanovas), I felt confident that she had many Soviet training secrets at her disposal. Those Soviets were famous for building the perfect human athlete and body. When it comes to knowledge and experience with sports, training, nutrition, and pretty much all things men want, just look to the Soviets, and specifically to the Bulgarians; I figured that Galya must have it all. In the spirit of the old Cold War days, I could "learn" from her.

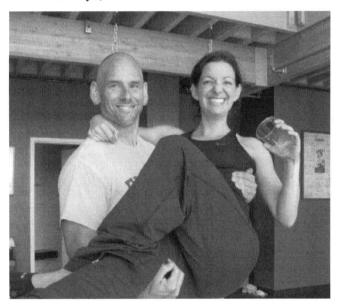

We had "met" online, before, so I already felt like I knew her, but over the course of several days, we discussed many things fitness related, and it turned out that we had very similar philosophies when it came to nutrition, training, and weight loss. While she had never been overweight, she had worked with hundreds of people who *had* been overweight, but aren't any more. I, on the other hand, had worked with only a handful of people, but I'd "been there."

For purposes of full disclosure (i.e., bragging), I have since married Galya, despite her outlandish claim that she has no secret Soviet secrets, I've seen her successes, so I know better. I will persist.

The two of us make a great team. I know what worked for me and the people that I'd worked with, and she was able to validate it against her own experiences back at her gym and with hundreds of clients. This stuff works, and together we have what it takes to make it work for you!

1

Life

You're busy with work. When you get home, the trash is piling up and the leaves need to be raked. You're busy with your wife, kids, and the dog. Your son wants to get an aquarium, and you know that's already enough to put you over the edge, so how are you going to find the time to lose weight?

How long have you been waiting? You've waited for the kids to be out of diapers and start to walk on their own. That's when you'd have the time, right? But still you wait to start. You're waiting for that gym to open close to work. You're waiting for summer so you can start jogging again, only to find that you're spending every Saturday watching the kids' soccer games. ...and now that the kids are older, your perfect gym time is being spent helping them with homework, only to leave you mentally drained and only capable of focusing on The Biggest Loser from the comfort of the couch.

You've waited, and while you've been waiting, your body has been doing what comes naturally – putting on fat.

There will never be "that perfect" moment to start. There is no perfect combination of circumstances that will come together to allow you to finally succeed and lose the fat, just like there's no perfect time to have kids, no perfect time to get married, and no perfect time to buy a house. I spent most of my adult life not losing weight, and every few months I'd look back and wish I'd started a few months (or years) ago. This repeated so many times that I lost count. More times than I can remember; it's a common theme.

The time to start is now. Yes, you think it's not the time because you don't have it in you to change life's circumstances. Life in upheaval? It probably already is. Whose isn't? Now it's time for more change? Please!

I've got news for you: the time to *succeed* is now. The time to *start* is now. How many more times will you look back at three months ago and realize that the time to start was back then?

Circumstances will not get better. Your success is going to be about managing your circumstances, not changing them. This book doesn't try to dramatically change your life, just dramatically change your body. It will help you analyze your life circumstances and manage them in a way that will give you the body that you want. You will transform without dramatically changing the life that you enjoy, but dramatically changing your results and your body.

Most diet and exercise books discuss two things, diet and exercise. Duh, right?

Why don't you start cooking low fat foods? Cut out all the fast food and restaurant dinners! Low carb? How is that going to fly with the wife and kids? They're all thin and trim already, so isn't it a cruel and unusual punishment to change up their lives just to make up for your expanded waistline and lack of willpower? Yep. Really, how much thought do diet and exercise books give to the life and meals of your family? Not a lot.

And what about exercise? You're already busy, so what is the prescription of three, four, or five trips to the gym going to do to your family life? How much time away from the wife and kids will running 10 miles a week cause? I mean, you can't stop working? You can't stop commuting? That leaves, sadly, cutting out family time. That's just not a good option.

The bottom line is that any dramatic changes to your life that would pull you farther away from your family, work, and responsibilities are doomed to failure. So, with that in mind, why not start with a look at your lifestyle as a whole and see what changes you can make to enhance your life and help you meet your goal to get back in shape?

We can't just look at diet and exercise; we have to look at life, too. What does that mean? Let's look at a partial list of things that comprise a typical day – work, play, housework, cooking, paying bills, washing the car, eating, yard work, exercise, shopping, homework, baseball practice, carpools, naps, and all the other things that fill up your day. These are all "life."

You can see that diet and exercise are on the list, alongside all the other important things in your day, but in the big picture they actually seem to rank pretty low in the scale of importance, don't they? What happens to your son's sporting future if you fail to go to the gym? Does your daughter's education suffer if you eat a burger and fries instead of making something healthy tonight? Nope.

Since it doesn't really have an immediate effect on today, it's pretty easy to skip the good diet and not go to the gym. Do that tomorrow and the next day and pretty soon you're back to old habits and buying yet another belt to outgrow.

We're back to looking at your lifestyle as a whole. Make no mistake, you won't succeed in your quest to lose weight and look the way you want without proper nutrition and exercise, but there's no reason why you can't make small changes that have dramatic effect on your body and actually increase your chances of success. So, in addition to diet and exercise, we're going to look at "life," too.

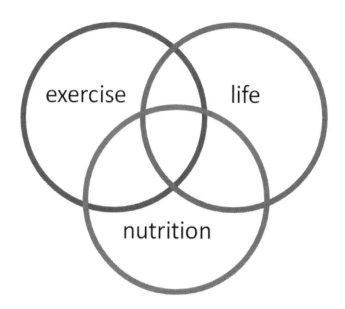

Three basic categories; life, diet, exercise. Look how they overlap! You're about to see how each not only has a dramatic effect on its own, but also affects the other two.

Keep reading, because it's time to start!

2

The Kickstart

What to do while you're reading this book

A "kickstart" is simply a way to get things started, whether it's a motorcycle engine, a complex corporate project, or even a new fitness program. You start *now*, fast and simple, and you're off and running!

How many times have you let a book linger on your nightstand – for weeks or months at a time – just *knowing* that there's life changing information in there? There's a book about organizing your life there; it's right on top. That one is sitting right on top of the book you bought last spring about starting your own garden. The book about running that marathon is just under your book on how to train your dog. Way down on the bottom is a book about procrastination. You just have to finish these books and then get started, because without knowing the whole picture, where do you start?

Can't I just skip to the end?

With some of these books, an easy way to quickly find out what to do is just to skip to the end. There's usually something back there where it sums up and repeats the steps, only in shorter paragraphs, simpler words, and using bullet points. Should I just skip all the details and tell you what to do without any good reason? I don't really want you to do that...

This book is going to create action - and your actions will be based on what *you* decide to do along the way. You will need all the details that I have included, because all of them will click at some point. This book does have a physical end, yes, but you will find the answers, and your fit and healthy body, along the way.

To kick things off, I'm going to have you do three simple things; log your food and activity, play around with a little exercise at home, and take some fish oil. Just three simple things, none of which will leave you hungry...

With the kickstart, you are going to have just enough information to start *today*, fast and simple, and then you're off and running! Instead of doing nothing while you read all the way to the end of the book, kick things off *now* with the Kickstart program, then it's back to your reading.

Logging your food and activities

Keeping track of things is going to be a big part of your success. This isn't some touchy feely journal or diary, so don't worry. I just want you to start writing things down. Print off the sample food log from our website (TheFitInk.com/ManOnTop), grab a spiral notebook, a composition book, or even the notepad or memo tool built into your iPhone or your Blackberry. The most important thing is to find a way to keep it handy and write in it often. If you leave it at home, but eat on the road all day, it will do you no good.

You can go into all the detail you want, but at the minimum, you should start with these three things at the top of page one – today's date, your body weight, and your pants size.

Optionally, you can also take some pictures or body measurements. Even though you might not like how you look right now, seeing your pictures change over time is a good way to know that things are working. I still regret not taking my own progress pictures (unfortunately, I hid from the camera in shame back then...).

After these simple items, you're going to start listing some things that you do every day, most notably eating and exercising.

Log your food– You don't need to change what you eat yet. Eat what you eat. Just write it all down. All of it.

For example:

Monday, May 7th

7:30a – 2 fried eggs, 2 sausages, 1 bagel, 1 packet of cream cheese, 1 packet of strawberry jelly, 2 cups of coffee with milk and 4 sugars

9:45a – Jelly donut, sprinkle donut

12:15p – Chipotle burrito with guacamole, large root beer

1:15p – 25 M&Ms

3:30p – Packet of peanuts

6:30p – Pasta with grilled chicken breast, salad, garlic bread, 2 light beers

9:45p – ½ a bag of microwave kettle corn, 1 can of soda

It's that simple. At this point, it's the writing that's important, not the calories, measurements, or exact foods themselves. You'll see later how to use this information to make some decisions.

Log your exercise – running, walking, cycling, weight lifting, baseball, etc.

Log your activities – cleaning, yard work, playing, walking the dog, etc.

Again, this early on, I want you to start becoming *aware* of what you do during your day; yard work, building a tree house, sweeping, taking out the trash, all of it counts.

Use the same log that you use for your food, and just write this stuff down.

7:00a – walked the dog, 45 minutes

12:00p – walked to Chipotle and back with Greg, 20 minutes each way

6:15p – trash, dog, water side yard, 30 minutes

7:30p – ~~Pilates~~ lifting weights, 30 minutes

9:45 – walked dog, 15 minutes

If you help around the house for an hour, just write it down as one thing. No need to detail everything in that hour unless it's really cool, like "I flushed a troop of badgers from the wine cellar." If you dusted the living room, washed dishes, took out the trash, and things like that, just write "housework" and be done with it.

Training – From zero to hero

There are a lot of fitness and training books in the bookstore, and almost all of them have the first few weeks of their training program dedicated to some training phase named "Beginner," "Break In," or something clever like "Phase Zero." I don't care for that, and judging by the number of questions I field from people asking if it's okay for them to skip it, they don't like it either.

It's not that you don't need some break in time, of course you do; going from zero to hero takes some ramping up. The great news here is that what you are about to learn in the next couple of weeks is going to stick with you throughout the program.

If you're not already working out, now is the time to start. Like I say on the virtual back of the book, there's no need to hit the commercial gym, you just need to train!

I'm going to blah blah blah on all this training stuff later, but at this point, just recognize that our ancestors didn't hit the gym to be strong and trim, they just *were* strong and trim because of their more active lifestyles. They didn't need to train for a marathon or spend hours in some basement gym to get fit, they just lived life.

Your training kickstart begins now. Today's workout is teaching you tomorrow's warmup *and* getting you fitter in the process! All of the exercises you learn today will appear again later. When that happens, you're going to be pleasantly surprised at how much better you are at the same moves!

Now, I will say that if you have experience with working out already, or you have been taking "a break," or are about ready to get back into it, by all means do it. We're not here to reinvent the wheel; we're here to get you back on track.

You guys with the experience – the former athletes and weekend warriors – are still going to find new things in our workouts, so at the very least give this thing a spin. Use our warmup for your own warmup, and fly through the circuit at least once or twice. If you find yourself feeling like our circuit was too easy and is closer to your typical warmup, then you keep training with your current program for now. Just keep logging your food and activities and we'll see you in the next chapter!

Workout basics

In the workouts and the workout log sheets you will see sets, reps, rest, etc. Here are some brief descriptions of some of these training terms.

Reps – Reps or repetitions are the number of times you perform an exercise. Reps will also help determine the weight you use. Always use a weight that is challenging, so that you could do no more than one or two reps beyond the prescribed number of repetitions. This practice, stopping even when you know you could get one or two more reps in, is called "leaving some in the tank," and helps to keep injury and overtraining at bay. Don't worry, grinding them out and muscle failure has been shown to *decrease* strength, not increase it!

Make sure you use more weight when you see fewer repetitions prescribed and less weight when the reps are high in number. When an exercise changes from 12 reps to 10, you also need to increase the weight used. Also, consider increasing the weight when things get easy and you feel like you are leaving three reps in the tank, rather than just one or two.

Sets – Sets are groups of repetitions separated with a rest break.

Circuit – A circuit is a sequence of exercises done in a row. A circuit can be done once, or may be repeated after a short rest period.

AMRAP – As Many Reps As Possible. Start your set and keep going until you can't do another rep with good form. If you feel like you could just squeeze out another one or two reps, that's the time to stop. Don't go until complete failure.

ALAP – As Long As Possible. Hold the exercise position until you can no longer maintain it, and your form starts to slip or sag. Don't go until complete failure.

Rest – You will rest a different amount of time depending on the phase of your program. Try to get close to the prescribed rest period, but don't stress about hitting it perfectly.

Glutes – This is short for gluteus, and is merely exercise lingo for the muscles of your butt.

The Kickstart Training Program

The warmup – this warmup isn't the standard "five minutes on the treadmill" that you'd get at a fitness center. Five minutes on the treadmill isn't a bad thing, but it warms you up for more treadmill time, not a full body exercise session. Our warmup is just enough to get your joints lubricated, your heart pumping, and your nervous system energized for the type of movement you are about to do. It will warm you up, but not wipe you out.

First, I will show you each warmup exercise, one by one, just to get you familiar with the movements. Don't worry, there will be a full list coming up, which should make it easy to follow along as you do your routine. I encourage you to go to TheFitInk.com/ManOnTop and download our blank workout log to record your routine and track your progress. . At the very least, get out a notebook or scratch paper and write these all down, along with how many of each exercise you need to do.

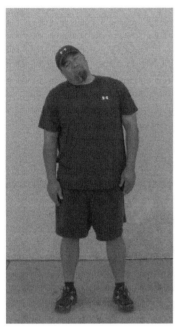
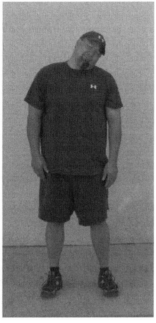

Joint rotations – Rotate each of the major joints (neck, shoulders, elbows, wrists, hips, knees, ankles) at least five to ten times in each direction, starting from the top down; gentle neck rolls, shoulder circles, wrists circles, bending left to right at the waist, rotating your hips, bending your knees and rotating your ankles.

About the models

I hope you appreciate our use of real people, rather than fitness models. Eugene and I had a great time taking these pictures, and we kept Galya challenged by forcing her to choose exercises that the "every man" could truly do!

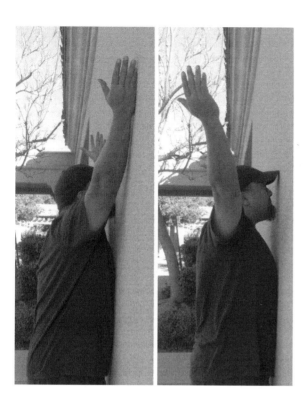

Face the wall Ys– Stand close to a wall and stretch your arms up and wide in the Y position. Use the muscles between your shoulder blades to bring your arms away from the wall, while keeping your shoulders down and elbows straight. Hold for a second. Return to the start position and repeat for a total of ten times.

Ankle mobility – Stand with your toes about six inches away from a wall and bring your other leg back. Shift your weight forward so that your knee darts toward the wall. If your knee can touch the wall, slide your front foot back another inch or so until you find it challenging. Repeat for ten reps on each side.

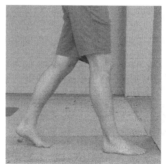 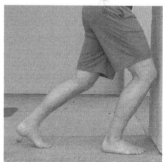

Split stance rotation – kneel down on one leg and put the other one in front. Stand tall and put your hands behind your neck. Keeping your elbows out, rotate towards the front knee and return to neutral, keeping your abs and hips in place. Repeat ten times and then switch legs and do ten more.

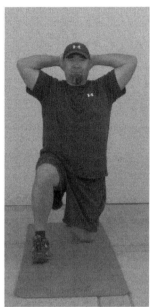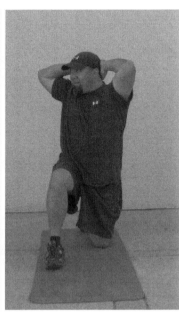

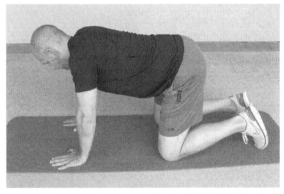

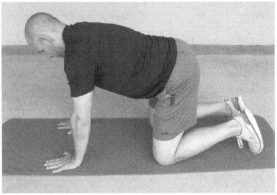

Pushups plus – Get down on your hands and knees and lock your elbows. Make sure that your low back is neutral (a gentle curve) and your abs are tight. Drop your ribcage down and let your shoulder blades come together. Keeping your elbows straight, push up with your shoulders so that your shoulder blades spread apart. Do ten of these.

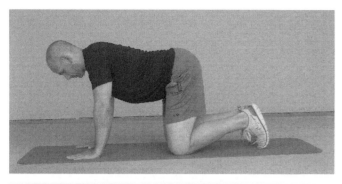

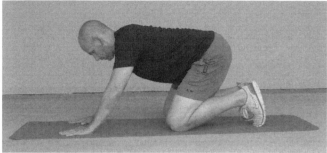

Rockbacks – Get down on your hands and knees and lock your elbows. Make sure that your low back is neutral and your abs are tight. Curl your toes under. Sit back, pushing with your glutes and keeping your low back neutral. If your pelvis starts to curl under, it's time to go back. Return to the starting position and repeat for ten reps.

Glute bridge – Lie face up and bend your knees. Squeeze your glutes and raise your hips off the floor forming a straight line. Do not use your low back. Lower yourself to the starting position and repeat for ten reps.

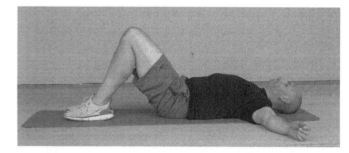

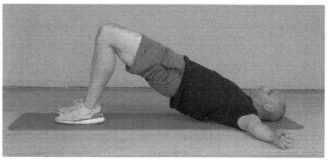

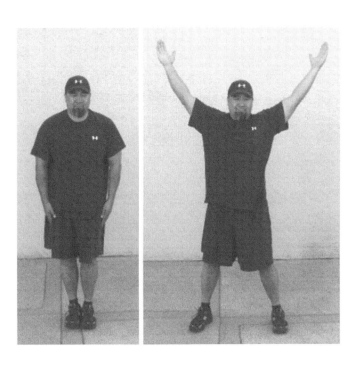

Jumping Jacks – Start with your feet together, hands at your sides. Jump and spread your feet to just beyond shoulder width, and simultaneously bring your arms up and together. Jump back to the starting position, and repeat for one minute.

...and that's your basic warmup, right there!

As promised, on the next page is the full list of warmup exercises, short and sweet.

Warmup

Exercise	Repetitions
Joint Rotations	10 per joint – each side
Face the Wall Ys	10
Ankle Mobility	10 per side
Split Stance Rotations	10 per side
Pushups Plus	10
Rockbacks	10
Glute Bridges	10
Jumping Jacks	1 minute

Warmup? Done!

The circuit – a circuit is merely a series of exercises done in a row. This first time, you might just do the circuit one time. If, at the end, you feel good and energized (although sweaty), you can repeat it up to two more times.

Like I did with the warmup, I will first show you each exercise, one by one, just to get you familiar with the movements. That will be followed by the full list, making it easy to follow along as you do your routine.

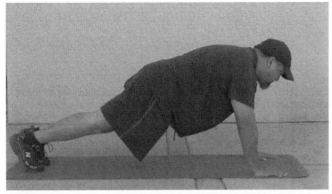

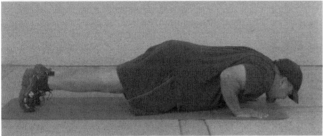

Pushups: Get in the classic pushup position, with your hands under your shoulders. Keep your abs very tight as you slowly lower yourself down, with your ankles, knees, hips, upper back and head in one straight line. Lower yourself until your shoulders are lower than your elbows and push yourself back up. Do as many as possible.

Do the classic pushup, if possible, but if you are unable to do any, you should do the Elevated Pushup, below.

Elevated Pushups – Put your hands on the bench, chair, or wall, slightly wider than your shoulders. Straighten your body over the ground, rising up onto your toes. You will be at an angle, not flat over the floor. Keep your abs braced the entire time. The tighter your body, the more pushups you'll be able to do. Lower yourself until your chest is an inch or two from the bench or chair. Keep your body stiff and straight. Push yourself back up, pause, and repeat for as many reps as possible.

Because this pushup is done with hands on a wall or chair, it is a good choice for those who can't yet do regular pushups. Elevated Pushups may also be used later as a way to do more pushups than you could normally do. Using a bench, low wall, or sturdy chair under your hands (instead of the floor) reduces the weight that you press with your arms and chest.

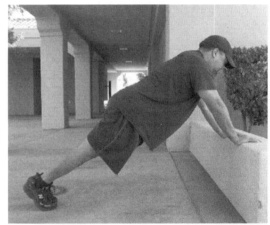

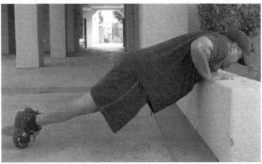

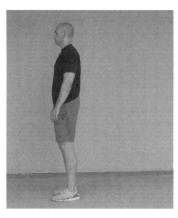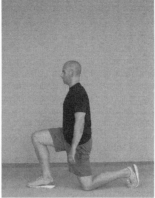

Reverse Lunges: Stand with your feet at hip width. Step back with one foot. Lower your body until your knees reach 90 degrees. Keep your back straight and your abs braced. Pause and push yourself back to the starting position.

I recommend that you do this exercise without any weight, but if you can handle the number of repetitions please grab a pair of dumbbells to make this exercise harder.

Wall Slides – Stand with your back against a wall and your feet slightly out from the wall. Raise your hands above your head with your forearms and hands in contact with the surface. Use your shoulder blades to pull your arms down the wall until your elbows are lower than your shoulders.

Over time, you will improve and be able to stay in better contact with the wall and be able to lower your elbows further. Don't force it and don't stick your chest out.

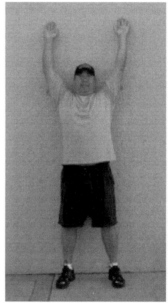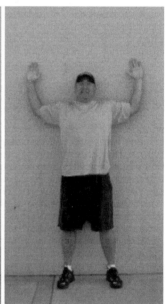

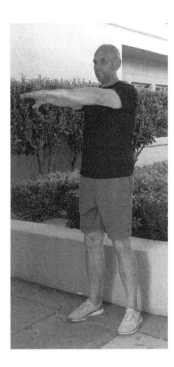 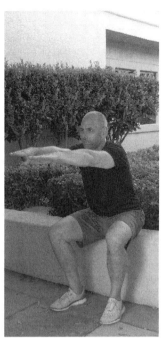

Chair Squats – You will squat down onto a chair, bench, or low wall. Stand with your feet about shoulder width, with your feet in line with your knees. Squat back and down, extending your arms as far as you need in order to counterbalance. Don't let your lower back round. Touch the chair and use your glutes to stand back up. Repeat for the rest of the reps.

Bent Over Ts – Assume a wide stance, bend at the hips, pushing your butt back and keeping your back straight. Drop your arms straight down with your thumbs pointing at one another. Keeping your spine neutral, pull your shoulder blades together, and raise your arms at your sides using only the muscles of your upper back. Hold for a second, then return to starting position and repeat.

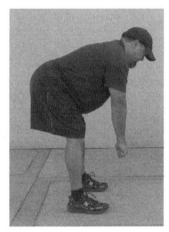 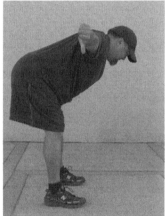

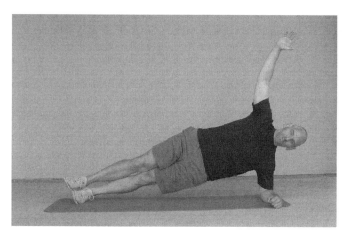

Side Planks – Lie on your side and place your elbow directly under your shoulder. Put your hips, knees, and ankles in line and push yourself up. Hold this position for as long as possible (ALAP) and then repeat on the other side.

If you are not ready for a full Side Plank yet, you can do them on your knees, as shown below.

Side Planks, on knees – Lie on your side, knees bent at a right angle, and place your elbow directly under your shoulder. Put your hips and knees in line and push yourself up. Hold this position for as long as possible (ALAP) and then repeat on the other side.

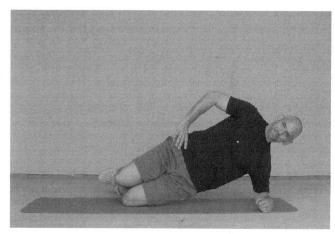

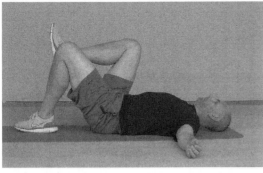

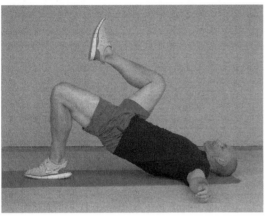

One Leg Glute bridges – Lie on your back and bend your knees. Lift your butt off the floor, squeezing your glute as hard as you can and making sure you are not using the back of your leg or your lower back to lift yourself up.

Bird Dogs – Get down on all fours. Relax your back and brace your abs. Extend your right arm and your left leg, keeping your low back neutral. Hold for the prescribed period of time, and then slowly lower your arm and leg under control. After you've finished all reps for this side, repeat for the other side.

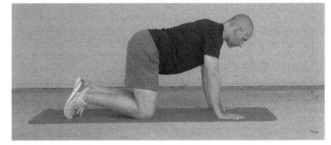

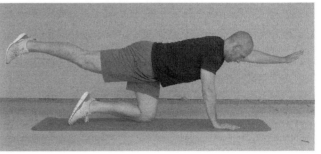

Kickstart Workout

6 Workouts

Exercise *Do In A Circuit* *Rest 1 Min*	Workouts 1-3 Sets X Reps	Workouts 4-6 Sets X Reps
Pushups	1-2 X AMAP*	1-2 X AMAP*
Reverse Lunges	1-2 X 10	1-2 X 10
Wall Slides	1-2 X 12	1-2 X 12
Chair Squats	1-2 X 12	1-2 X 12
Bent Over Ts	1-2 X 12	1-2 X 12
Side Planks	1-2 X ALAP*	1-2 X ALAP*
One Leg Glute Bridges	1-2 X 10	1-2 X 10
Bird Dogs	1-2 X ALAP*	1-2 X ALAP*
* AMRAP = As Many As Possible, ALAP = As Long As Possible		

Done!

You can stop if you need to, or repeat the circuit up to two more times after 2-3 minutes of rest.

How often should I do the Kickstart Training Program?

Two to three times a week for one to three rounds each time. Do this program while you continue to read the book. You can do the Kickstart Program for up to two weeks. When you get to the Fat Loss Workouts, you should be ready to move on.

When I train, how many times should I do the circuit?

The most important thing, at first, is to do the circuit at least twice a week. Do your warmup every time, then do the circuit once. Rest 2-3 minutes, then if you feel like you have it in you, do it one more time. Still have more time and energy? Rest again, and then do the circuit one more time. By the end of week one, you should be able to do the circuit twice. By the end of week two, try to do the circuit three times.

What if the circuit doesn't feel like enough?

If you really feel strong, energetic, and motivated, I encourage you to walk, hike, play, swim, or even clean the yard, rather than add another training session into your life. There will be time for more down the road, but it's important not to burn out. With strength training and resistance exercise, recovery time is as important as the time you spend exercising. Training is the muscle building blueprint, but rest is when the muscle is actually built.

What's not in the Kickstart

Yes, it's conspicuous in its absence. The D word. Diet.

Now is the time to get in the habit of logging your days and moving around more, not to start cutting this food and eating less of that one.

You bought this book to get things back in order, and I promised to help you with that. But another promise I made was to only change what you actually *needed* to change, and only as fast as you needed to change it. While there's little doubt that some diet changes are in order, now is not really the time, with on little exception; I want you to start taking fish oil.

But isn't fish oil part of "diet?"

True. You got me. Since you swallow it, I suppose I have to throw it into the diet category. But, I think of it more like a vitamin. It's just something you take every day.

Why take fish oil? I cover fish oil in detail in the nutrition section, but I do want to give you enough to go on, now. You may have heard of omega-3 fats, and that they may lead to fat loss, and better health. The most potent way to get these beneficial fats is to take them in the form of actual fish or as fish oil. Research shows that the addition of daily fish oil has been found to lead to fat loss *the very next week*, without any other changes. Isn't that enough reason to start now?

So, what kind of fish oil? I encourage you to buy at least one bottle of fish oil today, even if you know you can get it online for less. You have many choices where fish oil is concerned, as good quality fish oil is available at Trader Joe's, drug stores, and natural food stores such as Sprouts and Whole Foods. If you have a Costco membership, you can take care of your short and long term fish oil needs, today, as Costco's fish oil is inexpensive and potent: **Kirkland Signature™ Omega-3 Fish Oil Concentrate 1000 mg** – *1000 mg "Concentrated" Fish Oil w/300 mg Omega-3 Fatty Acids, 400 Softgels*

Other good brands are **Nordic Naturals** and **Carlson** in either capsules or liquid. Some are even flavored with lemon, orange, or even blueberry. This, however, may sound either more or less revolting, depending on your tastes.

For more information, check out the "Shop" tab on TheFitInk.com.

Keep it fresh

Always buy a brand of fish oil that's fresh, from stores that have a high turnover, and who store it properly (i.e., not in a hot warehouse or in the sun). When you get it home, keep it in the refrigerator or freezer to keep it fresh.

How much?

Studies show that even a relatively small amount of fish oil can have a tremendous benefit to fat loss, not to mention mood, heart health, joint pain, and general inflammation. The bottom line is that a small amount, taken daily can make you feel better quickly and help you lose weight faster.

Fish oil dosage

- Start with 6 capsules or a ½ tablespoon per day of a high quality fish oil, like the ones above or on our web site.

- After one week, you can increase the dosage to 12 capsules or 1 tablespoon if you have cardiovascular issues, joint pain, or depression, although fish oil is *not* a substitute for good medical care.

- Note: Be sure to check with your doctor if you are on blood thinning medication or have any issues with clotting, as fish oil can have an anti-clotting effect.

As you can see, you might end up taking quite a few capsules and may find the liquid to be more convenient, although the capsules have the benefit of letting you avoid the fishy taste.

That's it!

Log your food and activity, some light workouts, and fish oil.

It really doesn't seem like much, does it? It's not, but the whole of these three little things can easily add up to more than the mere sum if the parts. Just these three changes alone can kickstart your fat loss, lead to a better awareness of your diet and exercise habits, and leave you feeling better.

That's it for now, but please read on!

3

Your call to action

How to do something, and stop doing nothing

This book is designed to help you organize your life so it starts helping your weight loss goals rather than let you keep sabotaging yourself. It will take a few weeks to get everything together and feel like you are on top of your game, but meanwhile I ask you to do *something* that will take you in the right direction, rather than waiting for the perfect moment to start.

Life isn't about doing everything right, but about doing better than you did yesterday.

How to do something and stop doing nothing:

    Step One – Find out how life affects the way you look

    Step Two – Learn the skill of fat loss eating

    Step Three – Learn the skill of fat loss exercise

Just like any other skill, losing fat is a skill. You don't need boatloads of knowledge to get the body that you want you just need to have the right skills. Ages ago, our ancestors didn't need those skills, because their lifestyle guaranteed that they had a good ratio of energy in/energy out. It is only in recent years that our chair, computer and car bound lives have posed the need for new skills: the skill to lose weight through watching what you eat and the skill of knowing how to exercise. We have come to a point where we will either master those two skills or we will lose our ability to look good and be healthy.

Why is it that we can't just live our lives and stay in shape? Has our environment really changed that much? It's easy to get the concept if you compare your body to a rain barrel, like the ones that our ancestors used to capture and store water. Our ancestors' barrels were rarely all the way full, but they tried to keep enough in there for daily use. But, there was still room enough to be ready for the next rain.

That was then – when they did daily physical work, got plenty of sleep and rest, and ate high quality, whole foods, made from scratch. Today, we have a different story.

What would happen if every morning someone started pouring more water into your barrel (aka cheap, plentiful, low quality food) but no one was taking any out (aka too little sleep, too much stress)? Soon, the barrel would be full and start spilling over the top. Yep, this is now.

For most of us, modern life is "adding water to the barrel" constantly and not draining it off fast enough. Unfortunately, not everyone's barrel is the same size, nor is the flow of water coming and going at the same rate. There's no one solution that works well for everyone.

For instance, what if you are still living with your parents, having fun with your friends after you get off your low stress job, coming home to free food and a mom-cleaned house, and few cares in the world. Such a low stress environment means your barrel is never drained too far down and never gets too full.

What about your neighbor, who's juggling an executive job, has a wife who also works, and has four school aged children. His is a barrel that needs constant attention or there will be trouble!

You might want to jump right into this new lifestyle fully, following a complicated and restrictive diet, and exercising four times a week, but this would be a huge change, and a huge new stress, all on top of all the existing stressors in your life.

Your barrel is only so large, and this could be so much stress that it keeps you from starting or carrying on. You only have so much to give, and a big change is *not* what you need. An all or nothing mentality can ruin your attempts at achieving better health through being active. Each failure only leads to more stress, so the key is just *not to fail*.

This is how to do it – Put in effort where you can and don't sweat the rest too much. Put in effort where it gets you "bang for the buck" and don't waste your time and take risks with activities that don't.

All that matters is that at the end of the day you have just enough water in your barrel.

To know where you should focus your efforts, answer the simple questions on the questionnaire that follows. Once you have filled in the Life Questionnaire, you will know where you can focus your efforts in ways that will least interfere with your schedule, and once you find out what eating tips to use to alter your meals, you will be on the road to successful weight loss.

It helps to never forget that each effort stands alone, in everything you do; whether it's in your training or your eating, each effort is a chance to do better. Each choice you make programs your future body. Sit or stand? Double burger with fries or a bunless burger with extra veggies? Watch TV or play with the kids? Order a glass of water or have a third beer? It's your future body being made, right now.

Reality check

This is your reality check point. It will allow you to assess how your habits affect the way you look. Remember that the body you have today is the result of the accumulated effect of your habits. Some of the questions relate to diet, others to exercise and life - but they all matter.

Score each question with a number from 1 to 5. The lower you score, the more opportunity you have to change the way you look with the minimum amount of effort.

Feel free to use a notebook or sheet of paper, but remember that you will find a downloadable version of the form on our website (TheFitInk.com/ManOnTop), along with many other forms, logs, and tools. See Appendix 4 for more information.

Life Questionnaire

Eating Habits

Score each statement with a number from 1 to 5, where "never" is a 1, and "always" is a 5.

- I eat breakfast every day
- I eat protein with every meal
- I eat vegetables or fruits with every meal
- I avoid fast food
- I avoid sodas, juice, sports drinks, and other sugary drinks
- I avoid snacks
- I usually skip desserts

Work habits

Score each statement with a number from 1 to 5, where "never" is a 1, and "always" is a 5.

- I move around a lot at work
- I stand a lot at work
- I tend to fidget in my seat at work
- I avoid treats at the office
- My employer provides a free gym membership
- I am active on my lunch break

Free time habits

Score each statement with a number from 1 to 5, where "never" is a 1, and "always" is a 5.

- I play sports with my friends
- I avoid watching TV
- I wash my own car
- I make time for exercise
- I avoid drinking alcohol
- I walk for 30 minutes every day

Family habits

Score each statement with a number from 1 to 5, where "never" is a 1, and "always" is a 5.

- I cook most of the meals at home
- I play sports with my kids
- My whole family eats healthy
- I walk the dog every day
- I am always on top
- I do my own yard work
- I help with chores
- I do the grocery shopping

Now that you've scored your lifestyle habits, it's time to look back at your answers and focus on the ones that are less than a 5. Pick those habits that you can start changing immediately, rather than focusing on things that you aren't very likely to do now (or ever).

Every time that a habit moves closer to 5 you are getting closer to your efforts reaching critical mass, because all efforts count.

How likely are you to change a habit?

Whenever you decide to change a habit, ask yourself how likely you are to actually make (and keep) that change each day. Rate your motivation from 1 to 10. If it's under 7, you probably aren't motivated enough to make that change yet. Either change the parameters of the habit or pick another one that you're more likely to change right now.

Chandler, who's just getting into the program, decides that he's going to cook dinner every night, but when he rates his motivation, he realistically rates his likelihood of actually cooking every night a 5, which isn't quite enough. Chandler really likes the idea of making more dinners, so he decides to cook four nights per week, instead. When he rates this new goal, he gives himself an 8, which is safely above 7! Awesome.

You will be using this questionnaire about every four weeks to reevaluate your healthy habit progress. If you find that you are still in the same spot after a month, don't worry, just look at which habits you can do to move closer to a 5.

To motivate you to make positive changes or stick with them, let's consider what's in it for you to lose the extra weight or simply get leaner? You've already started looking at the habits that you have developed and are replacing them with ones that will aid in seeing a leaner, healthier you. Maybe you have a good reason to lose your extra pounds, or maybe you need to remind yourself why you are doing it.

Here are a few simple questions that might help you stay on track with your conscious and subconscious reasons for weight loss:

• What are you going to see when you achieve your desired weight? It helps to imagine yourself looking in the mirror, zipping a pair of pants that right now don't fit right, etc.

• What are you going to hear when you achieve your desired weight? "Wow, you look like you've been working out!", "you are hot!", "I'm sorry I didn't pay more attention to you in high school," "you've lost some weight, how did you do it?" etc.

• What are you going to feel when you are at your goal weight? Think of how your leaner waist will feel in jeans, how light you feel going upstairs, how your t-shirt will feel on you when it isn't stretched over that belly.

• What will you be able to do when you are lighter? Think of playing beach volleyball in just your shorts, being able to play with your kids without being out of breath, going out with your lean and healthy friends and feeling like you fit in, etc.

Goals

Like most people, you will probably find it easier to stay on track if you set specific goals and deadlines to your weight loss. I have seen that when people work with specific goals and deadlines, they are more likely to keep on track with their food and diet.

But, I don't have time to _____!

Walk – Take the kid, walk to the store, walk the dog, etc.

Workout – Get up early; don't waste time on TV reruns.

Cook – Make multiple foods at once, make all your lunches tonight.

Primary Goal(s)

In your notebook or on a sheet of paper, write down your primary long term goal or goals, such as "wear my size 40 jeans again," "lose 25 pounds," or even something like "have my doctor stop my medication for high blood pressure."

Supporting goals

Underneath your primary goal, list at least 6 supporting goals that will help you attain your main goal, e.g. make plan meals, do my exercises every day, drink ½ gallon of water, etc. These goals should support your primary goal, and will most likely based on what you discovered about yourself when using the Life Questionnaire and those habits.

Ideally, you want to focus on 1-2 supporting goals a week. If you are super busy, stressed, or a total mess right now, go even slower - you will get there one goal at a time, and too much, too soon is a disaster in the making.

	Chandler
	July, 7
	Primary goals
1	lose 40 pounds by my high school reunion
2	wear my Lucky brand jeans again by Christmas
	Supporting Goals for week one
1	Buy fish oil from Costco
2	log my food every day
3	take the Fitness Test
	Supporting Goals for week two
1	take fish oil every day
2	workout twice this week
3	
	Supporting Goals for week three
1	
2	
3	
	Supporting Goals for week four
1	
2	
3	

You can see that Chandler's primary goals are specific, achievable, and have a time element or deadline. His supporting goals are very task oriented, meaning that they are actions performed that will take him closer to his primary goal.

Chandler's primary goals were set early and likely won't change. His first two weeks' supporting goals have already been made, and you can see that they are the specific actions that will help him achieve his primary goals. His goals are focused on the present, and their combined effect will help him achieve his final results.

You can also see that Chandler's week three supporting goals haven't been done yet. Later in the book, I'm going to give you all sorts of ideas to support week three and beyond. In the meantime, take Chandler's lead, and write down your primary goals. Underneath them, write down the specific supporting goals that you're going to do to in the next two weeks.

Remember, when you set a supporting goal, always ask yourself how likely you are, on a scale of 1-10, to actually do it. If it's less than a 7, adjust the goal until it's a 7 or higher. You want to succeed, so choose goals that are achievable.

4

Success at your fingertips

How other people lost weight & kept it off

If you were climbing a mountain, it would help to know you are not the first one to even venture there. If you looked in the mirror and thought you could lose some weight, know that you are not alone. The fact is it's easy to gain weight and not that easy to lose it. Yet, there are people who wanted to lose weight and made it happen. To be successful at fat loss, you need to know where you stand and what needs to be done to get to your goal.

When Galya and I started writing this book, we wanted to give you no option of failure, so we interviewed many people who successfully lost weight and kept it off, and we found the following common denominators of success:

Five common denominators of weight loss success

1. The time is ~~never~~ always right

There's never going to be a perfect time to start changing your body. When you look at it, the body you have today is the result of months and years of choices. It just so happens they were choices that took you *away* from your goal.

We each only have so much energy to change, and sometimes we imagine that it's going to take huge amounts of effort to get fit and healthy. Shows like The Biggest Loser don't help, either. Just know that every day that we don't change confirms that huge misconception. One more day being your old self isn't just one more day in a body you are no longer happy with, but it's also a day in a body that's even more steps away from how you want it to be.

There are no perfect circumstances that need to come together in order to succeed. You eat every day, and you might as well eat the right things. You move every day, and you might as well do the best exercise for your body.

39

Every extra pound added before you start is an extra pound that has to come off later. You might feel like the time is never right to start, but because it *will* get harder if you don't, it's *always* the right time to start.

If you haven't started the kickstart yet, go back to that chapter and get on it! Be on your way to a life improving transformation! The decision to start might be tough, but the first steps in our program are not. Go read it and see.

Hey, if you're one of those people who *has* to start on a Monday, just practice until Monday. Start now, but count these next few days as a warmup. When Monday comes, you'll have hit the ground running, and you'll be a step ahead of yourself!

In each of the people we interviewed, something clicked at some point; they realized that they couldn't put things off until tomorrow anymore. They started "now" by buying and reading a book, immediately eating healthier, or going to the gym. It's not always the perfect start, but a start is always a good start.

2. Have a plan

Getting educated is what counts the most in fat loss. Many of the people we interviewed tried many things before they found what works best. Doing what works best for your weight loss goal equals results and results equal motivation to keep going. Many people waste a golden chance of permanent weight loss by making the wrong choice of a diet and making efforts that only temporarily improve their body.

It is common dietary mythology that fad diets lead to even greater rebound weight. While we don't advocate fad diets, I will say that it's not the diet that led to the extra fat down the road, but the lack of education that the diet provided. Sure, the weight was lost, but without knowing the whys and hows, and without learning the ongoing practices of weight maintenance, keeping the fat off was unlikely to happen; fad dieters just don't know how. They were not taught what it takes to keep the weight off.

This book will both educate you on the types of habits to change so you can eat a more sensible diet and move enough, plus it will teach you how to troubleshoot when things aren't going so great. We are going to teach you to lose weight, and how you can easily maintain your new body.

The people that we interviewed decided to take their weight loss education into their own hands. That didn't mean they didn't ask for or get help, but they took control. They bought a book like this one, joined a fitness forum (like JPFitness.com), and just started learning.

3. Have a next plan

People who successfully lost fat sometimes got it right the first time, but most times their success followed failures. Knowing that the last time failed is a primary reason why people don't try again; instead, they wait for the perfect plan or to hit rock bottom (sometimes it's rock bottom *again*).

Because the successful people we studied already had a next plan, they never strayed from their path. They had educated themselves on their options, and had a good one ready to go.

What if you find that your current method is making you miserable? What if it's simply not working? Take a lesson from these successful people, and never stop. ...and never stop learning.

One of the things that the people we interviewed had in common was channeling their voracious appetites for food into a voracious appetite for fitness or nutrition. They read books, listened to podcasts, and watched videos, all to learn more about methods that would ensure their success before they had a chance to fail!

4. Every meal counts & every meal stands alone

At some point, you will realize that each meal counts and empowers you to change the way you look. You will not change if you keep eating the diet that got you to be bigger, the diet that feels convenient, or many Thanksgiving sized meals.

You *will* change when you look at your plate and know that your good choices will get you there. Don't worry if one meal isn't perfect, but make sure at least 90% of your choices are in line with your goals.

If you fall off the bandwagon, get right back on it. If you fail at one meal, then follow it with another and another, pretty soon you will see yourself battling pounds that you shouldn't have had to battle in the first place.

The people we interviewed did not look at one bad day of eating and give up. They kept going. To them, every meal stands alone.

5. Permanent fat loss is the ultimate goal

You *can* achieve the fat loss you are looking for, but the key to continued healthy weight is to maintain the habits that got you there. This is why it's so important to internalize habits that make you happy, and allow you to maintain them long term. Those are habits that are designed to counteract the everyday negative effects of lifestyle: work, stress, bad nutrition, lack of exercise. Give yourself time to see which habits really work for you, and make those the base of your new lifestyle.

One of the things that we love about our system is that it allows you to find the methods that work for you, rather than shove our choices down your throat. Sure, we'll guide you and advise you, but in the end, you'll learn what works for you, where you need help, and what comes naturally.

Maintaining your new lifestyle should be fun and easy, especially after you get into the swing of things.

All of the people we interviewed lead different lives today, but none of them left their old selves behind. They still have their friends, and their families haven't shunned them because of weird dietary habits. In fact, their dietary and lifestyle habits are now probably pretty close to those of their naturally slimmer and fitter friends and family.

At this point you're probably wondering "what do these successful people know that I've missed all this time?" You might also be wondering why there was no mention of what to eat and what not to eat. Don't worry, that's going to come, but the most important take away from Chapter Four is that success comes from really wanting it. After you want it, it's important to plan, do your "research," always know your potential next move, be willing to learn from your mistakes and never let them destroy your progress and momentum!

It's almost time to read on and see how calories, activities, and different types of foods can make or break your success. First, I'd like to introduce our good friend John, who's an amazing success case, and the very first person we interviewed for this book. In fact, John was sitting right next to Galya and me when we first dreamed up the idea for this book, and deserves the #1 position in the success case spotlight!

Success in the spotlight #1

Once motivated, fat loss was easy for this guy

I've known John Gesselberty since 2004, and he's been a prime motivator for me ever since. John is a tell-it-like-it-is kind of guy. He doesn't pull any punches, and that's true whether it's giving needed advice or even when he's looking within.

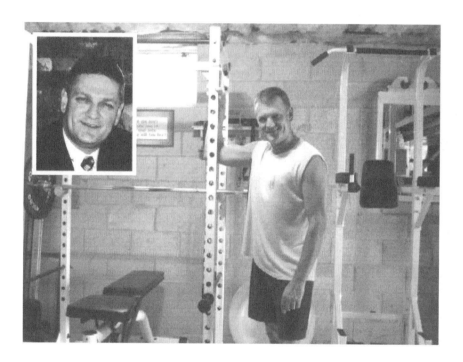

Years ago, faced with the prospect of buying bigger and bigger clothes, John instead made serious changes to his lifestyle. Within six months he went from 225 pounds down to 185. John has kept the weight off and only improved from there, inspiring and motivating us and others along the way!

John Gesselberty, 63 years old, and 55 lbs lighter

Roland – John, how old were you when you started losing weight?

John – Back then, I was 52 years old. I was shopping for new jeans. The 38s fit perfectly... and I remember thinking *&*&%^$^$!!!

John – I grew up as a skinny kid (28 inch waist at 30 years old). At that time in my life, though, I was very sedentary. I put the jeans back and said "I am not buying these."

Roland – What was wrong with your diet?

John – Home... dinner... TV... snacks. Chips and dip. I would snack on hot BBQ potato chips dipped in sour cream (a 7 oz bag of chips + 8 oz sour cream) in an evening. I was eating it because it was there and it was good.

Roland – What did you change to lose weight?

John – I started watching what I eat during the day, too. I was actively seeking what to do on the Internet. I was curious and hungry for results. I found fitday.com and I was floored with how much I was eating. 3500+ calories!

John – I set a time limit to not eat past 6 o'clock. The weight started coming off and I soon realized that I needed to exercise.

John – I looked for magazines, and found Men's Health. Got tired of the sit up thing and I thought I needed more balance. I was not athletically inclined, and needed something I could do alone, without the self-consciousness of someone watching what I was doing.

John – One day at Sears I got a universal training machine, the one that combines a few gym machines. I started exercising in the morning, got up at 4:15 and started my workout by 4:30, then I could relax, have breakfast and then go to work. This worked for me.

John eventually found his way to the world of good nutrition and weight training practices through Lou Schuler's book, The Testosterone Advantage Plan, learning about macronutrients and playing with them on Fitday.

John – I recorded all my meals for 6 years. I have recently stopped doing that, because knowing how much I eat has become instinctive to me.

Roland – What is your biggest challenge now?

John – Eating out is a challenge. I know that it will be a big meal because the calories will be too much. When I am out I eat healthy, but I know I will be eating something that's not great.

Roland – Any other biggies?

John – Eating at a relative or friend's house can be hard, but I usually take a very small portion of what someone has prepared. Large portions of the healthy things and small of unhealthy things.

Roland – Do you use strategies to reduce the damage of larger meals from holidays?

John – I restrict calories before and after a bad meal and I try to work out the day of eating. Whenever I come back from vacation I double up workouts... like a sprinting session at night.

Roland – What stops people from losing weight?

John – It's gotta be easy or its not gonna get done. You need to put your heart into it.

Roland – How much weight have you lost over these 6 years?

John – 225 to 173 lbs I leveled off around 173 and then with muscle gain I went back up to 190. I am very happy with the lifestyle that allows me to maintain my lower weight.

Roland – Did you read any books on weight or fat loss or training?

John – Testosterone Advantage Plan. I also got a calorie reference book. I could look things up when I was in restaurants. I bought Home Grown Muscle and I bought some free weights. Mike Mejia (of Homegrown Muscle and Testosterone Advantage Plan) taught me a lot about lifting. He used all different styles – power lifting, wave loading….pyramid…I started learning different set and rep schemes. It was a great program. The weights taught me a lot about attitude and overcoming.

Roland – Where did you get your information on training and nutrition when you were starting?

John – Mostly from the Internet and books.

Roland – What's more important in weight loss, diet or training?

John – It's the lifestyle. People fight over what system to choose, but there is not one thing….it's the lifestyle.

Roland – If you could go back and start to lose weight now, what would you have done differently?

John – I would have done more research early on and not fallen for the myths like spot reduction. I would have done more free weights. I respond very well to premade programs.

Roland – Why were you overweight?

John – Because I was sedentary and ate foods I didn't need to eat.

Roland – What are the three foods that you know are not good for you but you'd keep if you could still look good?

John – Pizza, chocolate…

Roland – That's two!

John – That's enough!

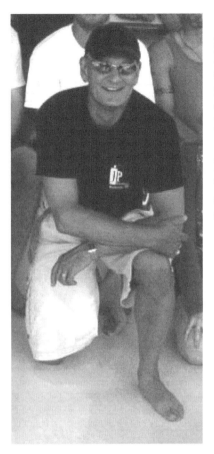

John Gesselberty is a regular contributor to and moderator of the JP Fitness forums, where he's known by his pseudonym, "Mahler," in homage to his favorite classical music composer. For more of his inspiration and motivation, look him up online on JPFitness.com, where he writes a weekly column "Mahler's Monday Morning Motivator."

Over the years, John has earned his position as the JP Fitness "Prime Motivator" by taking many of us under his wing, teaching us common sense, and inspiring everyone to deadlift, deadlift, deadlift! Let Chuck Norris have his Total Gym; John's weapon of choice is a barbell full of plates!

5

Calories are delicious!

You've heard that carbohydrates make you fat. You've heard that fat makes you fat. You might have even heard that too much protein makes you fat or that eating before bed makes you fat. Lately it's even been said that fruit makes you fat. All of this is true, because eating too many *calories* is what's making you fat, and all of those things have calories!

Calories *are* delicious; that's the obvious conclusion, because whenever you are faced with a food that's simply amazing and delicious, just look at the calories. I'll bet it's a big number. A big, tasty number.

How weight loss & weight gain really work

A calorie is a word used to describe a measurement of energy. It's used to show how much energy your body uses to move around, sleep, exercise, etc. It's also a measurement slapped on foods to show how much energy is stored within that food. Those calories are the potential energy that can be used by your body to move around, build muscle, create fat, and generally live life.

We talk about how many calories we eat and how many calories we burn, but we don't actually eat *calories*, we eat food, and as we just said, too much food makes you fat.

Calories aren't always calories

Sometimes calories are shown as kilocalories. You may see calories written as "Calories," "calories," "kilocalories," or even "kcals," making things pretty confusing. Technically, the upper case version of the word, "Calorie," and the word "kilocalorie" are the same thing. Why they would try to confuse you is anyone's guess. I'm sure they meant well.

In this book, on most nutrition labels, and when most normal people discuss them, they will mean kilocalories or Calories, despite the word that they choose or its capitalization.

Every day your body burns calories to keep you alive, breathing, moving, thinking. You eat to replenish the calories you burn with calories from food, and if you eat more calories than you burn, they need somewhere to go, and they end up stored as body fat.

Of course, that wasn't true for our ancestors, who had plenty of fat, protein and carbs in their diet. The bottom line is, while some foods are easier to overeat than others, it's the quantities of food you eat that make you gain weight. Food provides energy and if you don't expend that energy before or after it has entered the body, it will end up as unwanted fat.

It's really easy to eat a diet that piles on extra weight and doesn't let you lose fat. To illustrate it, let's look at a hypothetical friend, Chandler.

Chandler is a little overweight at 220 pounds, and he would love to weigh closer to 180. Chandler was nice enough to write down everything he ate and drank yesterday.

		July 9
8am	Grande mocha frappucino — 600 calories	
10 am	Coffee with milk and sugar, 2 cans of soda — 400 cals	
Lunch	bowl of chili and a steak sandwich — 1200 calories	
4p snack	2 mini packs of M&Ms — 400 calories	
7 oclock	garden salad, blue cheese dressing, BBQ ribs and a potato with sour cream — 1800 cal.	

Depending on how much he weighs and moves, he will burn different amounts of calories. Yesterday, he spent the whole day at this desk and burned about 2500 calories. He doesn't exercise at all and most of the calories easily get turned to stored fat. His total intake for the day was about 3300 calories, and this while he's trying to lose weight. If Chandler ate like this every day, he might easily gain a pound every week or so. This lifestyle is *exactly* what let Chandler's weight creep up over the years.

In order to lose weight, Chandler would need to lower his caloric intake dramatically, down to 1800 calories, so that he can be in a caloric deficit.

> *caloric deficit = eating less than you need*
>
> *caloric surplus = eating more than you need*
>
> *maintenance = eating just what you need*

Over time a daily deficit will add up and lead to pounds of weight lost. 500 calories a day will lead to about a pound of fat lost each week, since every pound of fat lost is about 3500 calories.

You might ask why we don't just tell Chandler to exercise. Won't that burn extra calories? You might be surprised to find out that exercise does burn calories, but not nearly as many as most people think. In addition, sometimes people get hungry and tired from all the exercise, and end up being even more sedentary *and* eating more, all without realizing it.

If Chandler started to run on the treadmill every night, he might think he's doing great, and for the first few weeks, he would probably even see weight loss results, despite thinking he's burning an extra 500 calories a day, jogging.

Unfortunately, studies show that he's probably only burning an extra 350 or so. Also, did you know that those cardio machines also add in the calories Chandler would be burning even if he was still at home doing nothing? That's the missing 150 calories, right there.

Most of us know people who have been jogging for years and haven't made much weight loss progress after the first month or so. It's often because they think they burn quite a bit more calories exercising than they actually do, but then also get tired, hungry, and burned out. In the end, they begin to do less and eat more, all without realizing it.

Chandler's fantasy jog? - 500 calories per day, or a 500 calorie deficit.

Chandler's reality jog? -350 calories per day. Extra eating from hunger? +200 calories per day. More couch time? +150 calories per day. Deficit? None.

Sounds hopeless, doesn't it? Don't worry, it's not.

One of the biggest benefits to exercise during weight loss is ensuring that calories that you do eat go to build the right stuff (muscle), and the calories you burn come from the right stuff (body fat).

You see, when you exercise, your muscle stores of nutrients get depleted, and when you ingest food, they get replenished. If you didn't exercise, most food would go to replenish exactly what you are trying to get rid of – your fat. In a bit, we'll suggest some simple changes that Chandler can make to his diet and exercise regime that will help him to slowly shed the fat he is so tired of. First, let's take a look at that guy we all know who eats whatever he wants and *never* puts on a pound of fat. The jerk!

Brian, the jerk, is Chandler's colleague at the office. Brian weighs 200 lbs and has maintained that weight since his late college years, when he played football. He managed to keep an active lifestyle and even though his job is sedentary, he spends a lot of time being active after work, going to the gym, playing with his kids and working in the yard.

Brian also wrote down what he ate yesterday and here is what we got:

		07/09
8 o'clock	vegetable omelet, coffee, milk — 700 calories	
10am	handful of almonds, protein shake — 400 calories	
12 pm	whole wheat chicken veggie wrap and an apple — 650 cal	
4:30	4 string cheeses — 300	
6	workout at gym	
8pm	steak salad with walnuts and bleu cheese dressing, ice tea plain — 1000 calories	

As you can see, Brian eats around 3050 calories a day, but expends about 3000 because of how active he is *and* because he has more muscle than Chandler. His diet and activity levels allow him to maintain a healthy weight with very low body fat. Most of the calories he eats go toward replenishing his muscle stores of nutrients or are simply burned off because he's so active.

You also see that he eats more like an athlete, and the foods he chooses are healthy and whole. This means the foods probably provide more satiety (are more filling and keep him full longer), so he is less likely to crave more food, not to mention sweets and sugary treats.

"Eating better makes it much easier to eat less." – Dr. Marion Nestle, author of Why Calories Count: From Science to Politics

How active you are can also determine what your body does with the foods you eat. If you sit all day and night, like Chandler does, there is a high chance that any extra calories will end up as belly fat. If you are active, like Brian, extra calories are more likely to go to replenish muscle stores and even build muscle if you're doing the right types of exercise.

Scientists have compared the effects of the same food on individuals who are active vs. those who are sedentary. Don't be surprised - they found out that the more you sit around, the more likely it is that a given amount of food will make you gain fat, even when calories are adjusted to ensure the same surplus. It seems that the hormonal response to foods and their calories alters with activity, so Brian has a better chance keeping the fat off than Chandler, even if he was to eat a less healthy diet.

It's not an exact science, since we can never know exactly how much we eat, how many calories we take in, and how much we burn.

Infomercials, daytime television doctors, and morning talk shows are frequently pointing fingers at mysterious ailments, and blaming failures on hormones, conditions, syndromes, and "metabolism." There's almost always some truth to these things, but they really only conspire to make us more confused.

It's not as simple as "eat less and move more," but it's not as complicated as the naysayers make it out to be, either. Simple solutions don't make good headlines, though, and they don't cause you to "tune in at 11."

The bottom line is that you must find a way to eat the right amount of foods and calories, and get your body into the mode to use them properly. Do this, and you will lose it and keep it off. Do this right and it will become second nature, just like it is for Brian and for all those other jerks who can eat whatever they want and stay skinny!

Understanding what your weight means

Now that you understand how weight loss and weight gain work, and the balance between how much you eat and how much you move around, it's time to show you what makes up your weight.

Have you even been on a diet, felt that your clothes were loose, felt that your exercise was working for you, making you fitter, lighter, leaner? Then stepped on the scale. ...only it hadn't moved.

You can literally see differences! The mirror is *clearly* showing your changes, and friends and family are all commenting, too.

What you experienced is commonly called body recomposition. You still weigh the same, but you have more lean body mass and less fat. Lean body mass is comprised of your bones, organs, water weight, and muscle, and is also known as your fat free mass. You store the rest of your weight as visceral and subcutaneous fat.

Visceral fat is the fat that produces those famously round and rock hard bellies that don't jiggle or give when poked. *Visceral* fat is the fat that sits between your organs and interferes with your hormones and metabolism, and often goes hand in hand with cardiovascular disease, stroke, diabetes and some cancers. Luckily for our health, it is also the fat that tends to be first to go with good diet and exercise.

Subcutaneous fat is the fat that you see and can pinch. It sits just under your skin, and is the fat that your body uses for insulation. It is less dangerous than visceral fat, but is also the type that hides muscle and makes you look like you need to lose some weight. This fat can also come off with good diet and exercise, revealing all that new muscle underneath.

Pound for pound, body fat takes up more space than the lean stuff. Bone and muscle are heavy and dense, after all. This is why you can lose inches around the waist, yet the scale doesn't budge; you've lost fat and gained some muscle, coming out ahead in almost every way.

How to track your weight

Once you start to make changes to your lifestyle and you start to lose weight, you want to be able to track your progress. You have several options to track your bodyweight, your lean body mass and your fat.

The scale

Pros – It's inexpensive and easy to use. It is also the one tool that you have used since childhood, so you probably already have a pretty good idea of what weight feels good to you.

Cons – The scale doesn't provide you with information about body composition, i.e. how much of your weight is fat and how much is muscle. If the scale isn't moving, and you don't know that you might have gained muscle, you may be disappointed with a plan that is actually doing you good. Your weight is also influenced by water/sodium retention and dehydration, bowel elimination, and hormonal fluctuations.

How to use it – Your weight can vary on any given day, depending on the food and liquids you had, the amount of rest you got, whether you recently exercised or not, and more. To help with this issue, don't weigh every day. Instead take your weight only twice a month, but on three consecutive mornings.

Weigh after you have been to the bathroom and while wearing minimal clothing. At the end of the 3 days, calculate your average weight. This is your current weight. Do this every two weeks to know how you are progressing.

Body fat scales

Pros – Body impedance scales try to calculate the percent of fat mass that you carry and provide a rough estimate of it without having to use special tools or pay someone to calculate the percentage of body fat for you.

Cons – Body fat scales give a range of inaccuracy that can vary between 3 and 10 percent. It's very hard to use them to accurately gauge progress.

How to use it – Use your scales in the morning, on an empty stomach, ideally after eating and drinking the same foods and liquids the night before. Make sure you wipe your feet with a dry cloth before each testing. Ideally, you want to test yourself as frequently as possible and use the average of three subsequent measurements as your accurate measurement.

There are handheld devices that work similarly, and both have the same benefits and drawbacks.

Measuring tape (girth measurements)

Pros – It's inexpensive and easy to take your girth measurements at any given site. It is a reliable and consistent tool.

Cons – Girth gives little information of the quality of the tissues. You may have gained muscle and lost fat and you would measure the same circumference.

How to use it – Measure the following sites: calf, mid-thigh, hip, waist, chest and bicep (relaxed). Sum up all the measurements and write down the number. Take measurements every two weeks, preferably early in the morning. Note that your waist measurement will often be the quickest to decrease.

Body fat calipers

Pros – They are the most widely used and one of the most accurate handheld ways of measuring body fat. After measuring skin folds on specific spots on the body, the numbers are entered into a formula. The result is the user's body fat percentage within a 3 percent margin of accuracy. Calipers also allow you to track local fat reduction in certain spots, so you know where your stubborn fat areas are.

Cons – It takes at least 100 measurements before you become good at pinching the sites in the same way. You may need special math skills, access to a computer, or complex charts to translate the skin fold measurements into your final results.

How to use it – Option one (recommended) is to find a good personal trainer who can do the measurements for you. Option two is to do it yourself. You may need help for the sites on your back and triceps. Whatever you choose, use a trainer or caliper kit that uses seven site Jackson/Pollock method and formula for the highest accuracy. Take each site measurement three times before you enter each number into the formula.

Take your subcutaneous fat measurement once a month, preferably before exercise and when your body hasn't been exposed to temperature extremes.

Before and after pictures

Pros – They are one of the most accurate ways to see muscle development, posture improvement, as well as fat loss. Even if the scale isn't budging, pictures tell the story.

Cons – You need someone else to take the pictures. This can be intimidating, but remember that the pictures will get better month after month. Those before and after pictures that you see on the internet all started with a before picture.

How to use it – Always take pictures in the same clothing, such as a bathing suit. Take them in similar light and surroundings. Take front, back, and side views.

Choosing your method

There are other, far more advanced, inconvenient, and expensive ways to accurately and reliably measure body fat, like the Bod pod or DEXA/DXA, however, you need something simple and cheap so you can track your results easily and frequently. Expensive trips to a lab aren't worth the trouble, as the exact numbers don't really matter. You merely need to know that you're making progress or that it's time to tighten up on your diet and exercise.

Choose a method that is easy and accessible to YOU. I have found a combination of the simple home scale, pictures, and the measuring tape to often be the best.

6

Nutrition

It's all about the food, baby!

Back in the "Life" section, I talked about how life, nutrition, and training work hand in hand. I talked about how life and its modern changes are leading to lack of exercise, and for many, weight gain. Now, here in this chapter, it's all about the food.

I don't want to get complicated on the diet side of things. I'll net this out. You can eat whatever foods you want and still lose weight. It won't be easy, but you can do it.

On the flip side, you can eat nothing but healthy foods and not lose weight. It won't be as easy, but you can do it.

I can do it, I'm telling you right now. I could be fat on healthy food. Seriously fat.

I have no idea how many diets you've tried over the years, much less how many friends you've seen fail at their own diet plans, but the odds are that you have heard of or tried the "eat less of whatever you want diet" AND the "eat as much as you like of X or Y foods diet." You've seen or even experienced a lot of failure. If you hadn't, you probably wouldn't be reading this book right now. Instead, you'd be doing one of those diet plans. Since you're not, welcome to our plan!

Unless this program was a cruel Father's Day gift or something like that, you are reading it because you have faith in our plan. Awesome.

If you're reading this book because it *was* a Father's Day gift, just remember that they love you, and they are just trying to help. You'll thank them later, right? Right. Now enjoy the book, read, and have faith. We've helped many people, and we can help you.

The D word – What does "diet" even mean?

Before I drone on too long, let's get this out of the way. I'm sure you've heard that popular phrase "don't call it a diet, it's a lifestyle." I don't really know what the deal is here, but this one bugs me. I'm over here rolling my eyes, if you can't tell. I know "they" mean well—that the word "diet" seems temporary, as in "let's go on a diet to lose 20 pounds." That does seem to imply that when the 20 pounds are gone, you can go back to your normal eating again. If you don't already know that this won't work, I'll be clear: it won't work. If you go back to your old ways, your old ways will put that 20 pounds back on, and for many people, it might be 25.

We obviously need a lifestyle change to keep the weight off, and the most effective time to start that is now, when the "diet" is starting. The time to figure out how to keep the weight off isn't at pound 19, but at pound 1. Now. Now is the time. The time is now. When is the time? Um... now.

All this is an interesting discussion, but no matter what the books and experts might say, I think we need to talk how people talk, not like a dictionary.

We can diet. We can go on a diet. We are going on a diet. We are dieting. Of course, when we're done, we are going to continue on our diet, because this is not a temporary thing, it's now our diet; it *was* our lifestyle change.

I've been "on my diet" for over 10 years now. I've been "done" for many years, but I'm still on my diet. How do I stick to it? I've changed my lifestyle and my habits, that's how. When people ask how I've done it, I typically say "I changed my diet."

Just think about the blank stares you'll get if you follow the advice of the "it's not a diet, it's a lifestyle" people. "Hey Roland, how did you keep that weight off?" asks Bob.

"Well Bob, I changed my lifestyle."

There will be a blank stare at the minimum, but maybe an eye-roll, too. And Bob *will* talk about you behind your back.

There is one time when "lifestyle" works better than "diet." Let me show you... "Hey Roland, how did you keep that weight off?" asks Oprah.

"Well Oprah, I changed my lifestyle."

Oprah leans forward, hand on her chin, eyes narrowed "please tell me more so I can write a blurb for your book jacket and propel you to stardom."

See how that works?

Back to reality. Feel free to use the term "diet." I use it and encourage it. When you discuss your dieting success, your lifestyle changes will still come up. In the discussion, it will become obvious that you weren't in it to lose 20 lbs, but to lose them and keep them off. ...via your new lifestyle. See?

From raw ingredients to packaged foods

A chapter ago, I showed you how our modern lifestyles have made it possible to do more with less. We do more work, with less physical work. The mere lack of exercise is an obvious problem, but it's not the only issue at play in our expanding waistlines. A major problem is the food itself. It's changed, too.

For simplicity's sake, let's only go back as far as the 18th or 19th century, when most of our ancestors were picking up food at the store. Our ancestors went to the store and came home with raw ingredients. Meat, eggs, milk, fruit, and vegetables. While there were bakeries for bread and desserts, I'm scratching my head to come up with many other premade foods that they could bring home. Pickles? Sauerkraut? You get the idea.

I think there are a lot of elements at play in there, and I can't single one out as the biggest issue. They each work together to cause an overall effect. Let's look at some elements of our ancestors' dietary lifestyles that helped them stay in shape.

• Most of our ancestors' foods were cooked and put together at home, from scratch. That means no preservatives, sweeteners and taste enhancers. You could easily identify those ingredients, such as corn, meat, fruits. Some of the foods you buy today have as many as 80 ingredients in a bite.

• Our ancestors were busy and active people. A couple of big meals a day were all they had time to prepare and eat.

• What about dessert? Judging by the "when I was your age" stories from my parents, grandparents, and great grandparents, dessert wasn't an every night thing. There was fruit on a regular basis, the occasional dessert on the weekend, and special occasions. Why no nightly desserts? Taking finances out of the equation, I'm going to guess that it was tradition and time that kept the dessert numbers down. Cooking several meals a day is already a lot of work, so making a dessert from scratch at the end of the day would just be more hard work. Today, we just keep a tub of ice cream in the freezer...

Speaking of the freezer...

• Our ancestors had no refrigerators or freezers. No coolers meant not cooking with "leftovers" in mind. I've noticed that when I cook knowing that I can put the rest away for leftovers, sometimes I go back for seconds or thirds. Pretty soon, there's not enough worth saving for tomorrow, so I just eat it. If you know you have to toss it, you don't make "extra," you just make enough for the meal. And no leftovers means nothing to accidentally overeat. Oh, no cooler = no ice cream. Let that sink in. No. Ice. Cream. You had to go out and get it, when it was even available.

• I already beat to death the fact that our ancestors were more active, so I won't dwell on that. I'll just mention that no coolers means more trips to the store. More trips is more moving around. More moving is more calories burned and more time where you're not sitting on your butt wondering what you can snack on.

Packaged foods and foods of convenience have shifted our idea of what a meal really is. Somehow I doubt that my grandfather would have been happy with a bowl of macaroni and cheese as his meal. Yet today, this side dish in a box (just add margarine and milk) is an acceptable meal? When did that happen? Where did the vegetables go? When did cheese sauce become a good replacement for real cheese or meat?

I'm sure some food historian can tell us exactly how these things played together and the sequence of events, but the bottom line is that it didn't happen overnight. One change and its societal acceptance led to another change becoming acceptable. It's been a nutritional vicious circle.

Packaged foods were cheap and easy, and the more they became acceptable, the more people bought. The more they sold, the sheer scale of it all allowed them to sell cheaper and cheaper. Another vicious circle.

A lot of this was driven by manufacturers' interests. Big profits can get bigger if they can find a way to make things cheaper and cheaper. Refined flour foods last longer on the shelf because the more fragile bran and germ have been removed. More fat and sugar keeps cookies and crackers moist longer in the box. Longer shelf lives allow them to make bigger containers for you to take home. No one buys a bigger container of cookies if it just stays fresh for a week. Are you kidding me? Now you can have a huge bag of cookies in my cupboard, where you can barely see the bottom. It'll stay fresh forever, seemingly. Based on the number of servings, it should last and stay fresh for weeks, but when it's empty midweek, you might have to pick up another bag! There's that vicious circle, once again.

With this new packaging and easy accessibility of food, our brains can't catch up. Being equipped with historical behaviors that protect us from starving is a problem when we suddenly find ourselves in a world full of plentiful food. We haven't had enough time to develop the skills that tell us enough is enough.

As the amazing eating behavior scientist and author of "Mindless Eating," Dr. Brian Wansink, says, "You will eat until there is no food left in front of you, or until someone has turned off the lights."

We live in a world where huge portions are thrust upon us

Do you realize that many restaurant meals can be more than double the amount that you should be eating at a meal? Restaurant meals can be huge! Not huge, wholesome, and nutritious, either; huge and full of calories, yet lacking in real nutritional value. The bottom line is that more nutritious foods tend to be more filling, have fewer calories, and are less likely to be overeaten. They will also tend to make you healthier; a nice side effect.

Let's look at some typical restaurant meals and their calories. Keep in mind that, assuming an ideal weight of 165 to 195 pounds, the average guy needs to eat about 2500 to 3000 calories to stay at his ideal weight. Chandler is our average guy representative, and weighs about 180 pounds. He would need about 2700 calories to stay that weight.

I'm sure you will recognize at least some of these restaurant foods:

Onion Blossom – 2700 kcal

Chili Cheese Fries – 600 kcal

Cheese Sticks - 360 kcal for two sticks

Nachos – 1800-2600 kcal

Potato Skins - 280 kcal for just two

Wet Burrito - 1600 kcal

Let's take the first food as an example: the onion blossom. Let's assume our friend Chandler is going to share it and just eat half of it. That onion blossom is 2700 calories. Half is 1350 calories. Chandler gets 2700 calories for the day, remember? That's half of Chandler's food for the day, right there. Before dinner!

I don't think anyone thinks that these things are actually healthy, but I doubt most people realize just how bad they are for your waistline. Take Chandler's lack of knowledge, brought on by some denial; add in some procrastination, and one morning you're unable to button the fat jeans you just bought last month. Oops. Yeah, I guess those onion blossoms are bad…

So, that's just your appetizer, bring on the meal! Mmm… 1350 calories of oniony, fried goodness just went into your belly. By all rights you're not actually hungry anymore. But, over time, you've conditioned yourself to overeat, so you do want to eat more. Bring it on! So, you order up and overeat. In some cases, it's overeating in calories, and in others it's overeating in calories and volume. Think "eating pants," and you'll know what I mean.

One of my kids' favorite restaurants is a major chain whose decor is that of a mining camp in California's Gold Rush days. The food is pretty tasty and last time I went, I found a ton of healthy choices there. They had stew, for instance, that included beef, potatoes, carrots, onion, peas, corn, etc. Each ingredient is arguably healthy enough on its own, but then you have to consider the thick gravy and the sourdough bread bowl. Once you've ordered, you might be in for a big surprise – or not, since you probably went there because you *want* the huge portions… If you haven't figured out the surprise, it's only that the serving of stew is immense, and the bread bowl is gigantic; big chunks of beef and veggies, potatoes, gravy… shall I go on? No? You get it? It's big. It's probably enough food for your family, calorically speaking. But, it's on *your* plate and *you* are going to eat it…and you do.

Why are portions so big these days? I have some ideas, and you probably do, too. Off the top of my head, I'd say people who overeat want to overeat in a cost effective way. It doesn't cost much more than a few cents for the restaurant owner to add more gravy and potatoes, and those bread bowls are cheap, cheap, cheap! Soon, you're eating 400 extra calories for only two dollars more and coming back week after week. There could be other reasons, but those are discussions for Internet forums and blog posts. The bottom line is that we have to live in a world where huge portions are now thrust upon us, and we must find a way to deal with it or somehow keep buying larger and larger pants.

Now some purists will argue that we are fat because restaurants use cheap food and nasty ingredients that are inherently fattening and unhealthy. They are often right about the unhealthy part, but cheap foods and nasty ingredients, in and of themselves, don't necessarily make us fat. I'm a big fan of healthy foods, but let's make sure we don't confuse the issues. I can eat "clean foods" and get pretty fat; it's just not as much fun.

Why "clean eating" isn't enough

Around the Internet, the popular kids say that eating clean will get you there. What or where is "there?" Doesn't matter, "there" is having less fat, running a marathon faster, piling on muscle without putting on any fat, lifting harder, lifting longer, whatever. This is freaking awesome! All you have to do is eat clean and "there" is all yours! But, the only problem is that it's not true.

The first problem is the definition. What does it mean to eat "clean?" It's different for everybody. What if my "clean" is your "dirty?" Without trying to judge, I'll give you a few "for instances."

There are people in the world who try to eat close to how paleo man probably ate. These paleo types avoid grains and starchy carbs, sugar, and often even certain fruits and veggies that either weren't available in the caveman cave-stores or were vastly different back then. To these people, a bowl of oatmeal is anything but clean eating.

There are others who consider clean eating to be a bowl of oatmeal, with ground flax seeds sprinkled on only *after* cooking the oats, so as not to ruin the bioavailability of the omega-3s in the flax seeds. Protein powder should be stirred in after cooling the oats, so that the protein is not denatured.

Yet another group says that to eat clean, meat must be lean; fat is fine, but only if it's added separately to the meal in the form of olive oil. Bread is fine, as long as it's whole grain and consumed in the two hours after a workout, during which your body is prepared for and ready to use carbs efficiently.

All of the above scenarios can be considered eating "clean," but none are clean to everybody. Eating clean is really just a set of rules laid down by somebody who thinks their own style of eating is healthy. Like I said before, healthy doesn't always make you thin; it just may make you healthy (or healthier).

Eating according to someone's Rules of Clean Eating might make it harder to overeat or easier to diet, but only if you don't feel like overeating those foods. I, for one, can eat A LOT of oatmeal. In fact, I need a lot of oatmeal just to be satisfied while I'm eating, and even then, it doesn't keep me full for long. After the oatmeal, I'll probably have to "eat clean" again in just a little while. So much for clean eating keeping the weight off, right?

After all this, you might think I'm against clean eating, but I'm not. I encourage clean eating, but it's not the secret to fat loss, lack of fat gain, lean bulking, or high performance in sports. It has benefits, but it's not the Holy Grail.

Let's take a look at some benefits, before I talk you out of eating clean.

• Clean eating promotes better health – clean eating foods tend to be closer to the natural versions, have less added sugar and fewer preservatives, healthier fats, and more vitamins, minerals, and fiber. They tend to promote healthier levels of cholesterol and keep high blood pressure away, too. If you are genetically predisposed to developing diabetes or hypertension, you are less likely to develop them if you avoid most man made foods.

- Clean foods tend to be harder to overeat – not impossible, just harder. Calorie per calorie, they take up more room in your stomach than processed foods do, and they take longer to digest. They are also harder to chew, so you eat them more slowly. The veggies that replace or displace some or all of the pasta, rice, potatoes, and bread are far less likely to be binge eaten, and even if it happens, they are far lighter in calories than what they replace. Fruits are lower calorie than almost any dessert or snack item, are higher in water, take longer to eat, and are far harder to overeat.

- You mentally feel better about eating clean – it's one of those circles again, but hardly vicious, in this case. You eat healthy and give yourself that virtual pat on the back, so you continue to eat healthy. You eat less, so you're less bloated, less gassy, and feeling great, so you keep it up. You probably lose weight, fat, or inches, so you give yourself a little cheer and then keep up the good work.

- Clean eating tends to encourage people to cook more – or even learn to cook. There aren't too many clean foods that come prepared, or in boxes labeled "instant." Clean foods don't make themselves, but it's not all that hard, either. Cooking your own food gives you control over taste, quality of ingredients, and calories. Later in the book, I am going to be giving you some easy to prepare recipes for your own meals, and even some that the whole family will love. They won't even know it's healthy, so don't worry. It will be easy stuff that is also manly like chili and cowboy food, so relax.

- Clean eating gives you fewer cravings. Many people believe that our bodies tend to expect a certain level of nutrition, vitamins, and minerals from our foods. Junk foods, boxed, and processed foods simply don't provide the levels that nature has led us to expect. As a result we may end up with more cravings, and subconsciously seeking out foods just to get more of the vitamins and other things that we're not getting in our poor quality foods. Wouldn't it be perfect if we craved veggies, chicken, and fruit? But you know that's not going to happen all that often. More likely than not, the cravings are going to have you opening the cookie jar or looking for the ice cream. That's not good...

Of course, there are more good reasons to "eat clean," like fewer blood sugar spikes and crashes, less insulin resistance, better heart health, clearer skin, and feeling generally better, blah, blah, blah.

Clean eating does help with long term good health, and it tends to make fat loss or weight loss more manageable and sustainable. The two can be intertwined, so there's good reason to eat clean.

Every meal stands alone

At first glance, you might think that I'm doing you a disservice by telling you the truth here, but let me show you why I'm doing it. It's not that I think that everyone needs the truth put in front of them. I don't. I believe heartily in the placebo effect, so when it works, I'll let you wallow in your own delusions as you get thinner for all the wrong reasons. But, right now, I'm thinking of you and your long term success. Here it comes...

By all means DO eat healthy, but don't let a bad choice ruin your diet or your progress. What I mean is this: an onion blossom (um, not "clean" at all) is not the end of your dietary progress. If you could find it in yourself to eat only one tenth of that blossom, you'd be just fine. When I demonized the onion blossom earlier, I called it out for its 2700 calories, so one tenth of that is 270 calories. While this would make a very unsatisfying appetizer, since that tiny portion of the dish is, as I just said, tiny, the actual makeup of the food will not stop fat loss. Too many calories stop fat loss, not onions, breading, oil, or a mysteriously delicious dip that may or may not be Ranch dressing. Too many calories are much worse than too many unhealthy ingredients where losing fat is concerned. This is an extreme example, since it's unlikely that you will eat one tenth of something like an onion blossom, but the principle is good with pretty much any food.

We live in a world where we are exposed to and offered all sort of foods that are not "clean." Sometimes, that's all there is to eat, but you always have the choice to eat less than what you are served. If you do that – eat less – you will do great, good, or at least better than if you chowed down on the whole plate of badness. My point is that there is room for bad foods, and they are not the end of the world OR your diet.

Like I said before, it tends to be harder to stay on track with too many bad foods, so I find it better to keep as clean as possible, when possible. But, if calories are kept under control, you can continue to do well in the fat loss department, some unhealthy choices or not. Again, I'm not advocating bad and unhealthy foods, but if you totally avoid the foods you love, eventually you might find yourself binging on the very foods you've been avoiding, or totally giving up your new diet or lifestyle out of the sheer misery of never having your favorites.

Hopefully, you eat less food when you eat bad food, but what if you don't? What if you overeat? This is important. Pay attention. Ready?

It's not the end of the world.

Very often, a binge or overeating "incident" can be the end of a diet. Once you slip up, the urge is often to simply give up. Don't.

Yes, you did a bad thing, but here's the deal. Every meal stands alone. Say it.

Every meal stands alone.

Every meal stands alone.

Every meal stands alone!

Every meal stands alone!

Got it?

Good.

When you overeat at a meal, the urge is to throw up your hands and give up. Bring on the goodies! Sack your workout for the day and let your diet go down the toilet! With luck, you'll wake up the next morning, frustrated at yourself, but ready to get back on track.

Getting right back on track with your diet sounds really good, and it's very mature to turn yourself right around and get back on your program (good job, buddy!), but we're not always that mature. Sometimes we end up taking the rest of the day off when breakfast was the bad meal. Sometimes, a Friday night happy hour with friends leads to starting off your Saturday with a bad breakfast choice. That can lead to a bad lunch, and then pretty soon it's Sunday and you're looking back on an entire weekend of dietary debauchery.

One bad meal isn't all that bad, but you can do a lot of damage over an extended period of time. The meals where you're not following a good diet can be seriously damaging to your health and waistline, which is why you're reading this book in the first place.

You can do so much damage in a few solid days of overeating and junk food that you may totally halt or reverse your progress. If it's bad enough, your mistake could cost you a week's or month's worth of weight loss and make you very, very frustrated. If you get frustrated at yourself for this too often, and you might just give up. Do you really want to hit rock bottom again to get back on your plan?

Every meal stands alone.

"Every meal stands alone" is a good mantra to use to snap yourself out of a binge or jump back into it when you overindulge in a meal, but things will go even better when you've made allowances in your plan to include some less than optimal foods. You should find a way to eat your favorites here and there, or else you risk becoming demotivated and falling *completely* off the wagon.

If it's part of the plan, it's not cheating

This is not an Ashton Kutcher quote, but good dietary planning advice. Most sensible diet programs recommend making the "cheat" or "free" meal a part of your official plan – usually just free meals, but sometime even free *days*. There are very good reasons to recommend a type of free or fun meal.

There can be physiological reasons for periodically eating some of these foods. For instance, very low carb diets, for a long period of time, can affect hormones and mood negatively. Adding more carb rich foods can keep your metabolism from crashing and hormones in check.

Most diets acknowledge the psychological value of one's favorite foods not being totally banished from the diet. When you can never eat a favorite again, it's pretty grim.

Let's take a look at a few successful strategies to work free meals into a program. You will see that you can take quite different approaches and still be successful.

The Precision Nutrition System, one of the most successful programs out there, recommends about 10% of meals or "feeding opportunities" be considered free meals. If you eat 28 times per week, then you get 2.8 (let's call it 3, because I'm feeling generous) free meals per week.

Be careful, even with carefully doled out cheat meals, you can still blow it if you eat three meals of lasagna, wine, and cheesecake, and wipe out any caloric deficit that you had from the other 25 meals. You still have to be smart about it!

Other programs can be quite restrictive most of the time, then quite liberal when it comes time to kick up your heels. If you are very strict all week, there may be room for an entire day or weekend of eating what you will. A low carb diet, for instance might be low carb Monday through Friday, and then allow sandwiches, potatoes, and pasta, come Saturday.

Beware, you can still undo all your progress by eating too much of your low carb foods during the week, then living large on the weekend! Even though low carb diets may have some easy fat loss advantages, if you lose one pound during the week and gain a pound back on Saturday and Sunday, you are back to square one on Monday. ...and frustrated.

Other plans might have you plan out more liberal meals or ingredients, as long as they fit into your calorie plans for the day or week. These meals are not as free, but they are certainly more liberal than those during the rest of time.

One example is being allowed 200 calories of sugary foods per day, eaten whenever you like. It can be part of your nightly dessert, as a couple of cookies with lunch, or sugar added to foods like oatmeal and yogurt. You don't get a cheat meal, but free calories to 'sprinkle about" as you see fit.

Keep in mind that this method might feel pretty restrictive to people who have decent self-control. Some people want a little time to eat without counting and measuring, and extra or "free" calories aren't enough freedom. It does tend to help those people who might be prone to a binge when they get the opportunity to eat whatever they want. We are all different.

From personal experience, my cheat meals work best when I mentally try to keep my overall day on track. I might even have to look at my whole week to make sure I accommodate all the extra calories. At worst, I fall back on the mantra from the previous section; "every meal stands alone."

As we know from experience, it's easier to stay on a sensible diet than it is to start one. That is why we don't want ever get off plan. Ensuring that we get enough freedom in our plan is one way to make sure we don't lose motivation. A very Spartan diet, which looks like it's going to last forever, is a sure way to make sure your diet fails. **Find a way to fit the foods that you can't live without into your diet, so when you do eat them, you don't feel like you've failed.**

But wait, there's more!

Most diets out there make some pretty big claims. In addition to helping people lose fat, they also commonly claim to improve cholesterol, lower blood pressure, promote insulin sensitivity, improve sex drive, increase concentration, energy, sleep, and almost everything else that ails us! All of these claims, rolled into one product? This seems too good to be true! How is this possible?

It turns out that most non-extreme diets seem to have many of the same health benefits, yet they take such different approaches that it seems very unlikely that they could have such similar effects on our health. ...yet, they do.

Super low carb diets claim big health benefits, yet so did the popular low fat diets that have thankfully lost so much steam over the years. Vegetarian? Paleo? All have been shown to improve x and reduce y, to great success! How is this all possible? What is the healthiest diet? We asked our friend Alan Aragon, nutritionist extraordinaire and master of nutrition and fitness research, for some help to break down and digest this question.

According to Alan, there are some common denominators of the healthy and successful diet. We call them "healthy diet tenets" because "common denominators of the healthy and successful diet" is really long and hard to type. Plus, if Alan copyrighted his term before we published this book, we would have been screwed!

A while back, over several cups of coffee, Alan, Galya, and I came up with this list of common aspects of good diet and health improvement plans. You'll see that it might not always be merely what you eat or don't eat that improves your health, but how much you eat, and your level of activity. Let's take a look.

Healthy diet tenets

1. Calories

Eating only what your body needs seems to be key, according to Alan. When you overeat, particularly for long periods of time, your body has to work at keeping you healthy. Constant overeating, particularly when it comes to the "bad stuff" wreaks havoc on your body's systems, leading to chronic inflammation, insulin resistance, dramatic blood sugar highs and lows, and much more. Our body is a complicated machine, capable of working with a variety of foods, but when you challenge it for a long period of time it can only take so much. Eventually, your health shows the damage right along with your waistline.

To quote Alan Aragon: "A hypo caloric state in and of itself has been seen to impart lipid improving effects regardless of changes in dietary composition!"

Translated into English, this means that when you are overweight and begin eating fewer calories, and thus lose weight, health markers typically are seen to improve – bad cholesterol, triglycerides, blood sugar, uric acid, etc. – regardless of changes in actual foods eaten.

2. Fats

Dietary fat is not unhealthy, and is critical for good health. Luckily, the 80s and 90s are gone, taking the low fat craze with them. With those days gone, it's time to embrace the good things that fat has to offer, while keeping in mind that while fat is not inherently bad, there can still truly be *bad fats*.

We're going to start with the bad fats because it's often easier and more important to limit these bad ones than it is to focus on adding *more* good ones. Still, there are good reasons to add certain fats, as you will soon see.

Trans-fats

As we're about to show you, there are very few fats that are actually bad, but trans fats *are* bad and should be avoided. Trans fats have been in the news a lot in the past few years, so you're probably already familiar with what they can do to your health. The TV and Internet news outlets have informed us that the consumption of trans fats increase the risk of coronary heart disease, raising levels of our "bad" LDL cholesterol and lowering the levels of the "good" HDL cholesterol. They are just bad news. Trans fats are found in many packaged foods, shortening, margarine, and spreads. You can identify them on an ingredients list when you see oils and fats that are listed as "hydrogenated" or "partially hydrogenated." In addition, ingredients such as shortening and margarine can contain trans fats, and are best avoided.

Omega-6 fats

These polyunsaturated fats are often lumped into the good fat category, and it's true, technically, that they are good, but only when they are balanced out by a good amount of omega-3 fats. However, most modern biochemists and nutritionists tell us that today's diet contains too many omega-6s and not enough omega-3s, making it hard to naturally balance these fats out.

Too much of the 6s and not enough of the 3s (the imbalance), leads to a sort of systemic and chronic inflammation throughout the body. Over time, this inflammation seems to lead to all sorts of nasty health conditions, like heart disease, joint pain, arthritis, and immune system deficiencies.

There's almost no stopping omega-6s from being a huge part of your diet, since corn oil, soybean oil, and the generic sounding "vegetable oil" are rich in this type of fat. Whatever else you do, try to minimize your consumption of these fats, not only avoiding those specific oils, but foods that contain them, such as dressings, and other packaged foods.

Oh, remember the first bad fat that I talked about? Trans fats? Well, those are almost always made with oils and fats that are rich in omega-6s anyway, so avoiding both is often a two birds, one stone sort of deal.

Those two fats (trans fats and omega-6s) are the "bad fats." I know, I know I left out saturated fats, but bear with me... They aren't bad. Be patient.

Omega-3 fats

These fats are the flip side of the omega-6 fats from a paragraph or two ago. Not only do we get too many of the 6s, but most of us don't get nearly enough of the 3s. The best source of omega-3s is primarily fish and fish oil, despite the marketing behind many products containing other, lesser sources of omega-3s. A good fish oil supplement, algae based omega-3 supplement, or eating fish like salmon or mackerel goes a long way toward maintaining your good health.

On those "lesser" sources of omega-3s, we'll say this: manufacturers of food products are quick to capitalize on health trends, whenever possible, and omega-3s are no exception. While it's true that things like walnut oil, sesame oil, and even soybean oil contain some omega-3s, the amount is pretty small. To make things even worse, the amount of omega-6s that they contain is so huge that it's actually making things worse, despite the presence of the 3s. Remember, it's not just that we need more omega-3s; we also need less omega-6s.

Some seeds, such as flax, are rich in omega-3s and lower in omega-6s, but they are still not the best choices for you in a quest for more omega-3s. Our bodies would need to convert plant sources of omega-3s (ALA) into a form that we can actually use (DHA and EPA). This conversion rate is really low (20-30%), so it would take a ton of flax to get a decent amount. It's just not a practical source. This is not to say that you can't eat these seeds, as they have plenty of other health benefits, but if you're looking for more omega-3s, look to fish, fish oil, or an algae based omega-3 DHA/EPA supplement when possible.

Monounsaturated and saturated fats

Once you've got your omega-3s higher and your omega-6s and trans fats lower, we're left with monounsaturated and saturated fats. These two fats will pretty much take care of themselves by managing the other fats. A healthy diet contains a mixture of all of these fats, and since they are everywhere, it's often easiest just to take strides to limit the ones that are specifically bad and focus on eating the good.

That being said, when you see favorite fats and fatty foods like olive oil and olives, coconut and coconut oil, avocados, and most meats and dairy products, rest assured that the fats in these items aren't bad for you. In fact, they are pretty good for you. With animal products, they will be even better if they come from grass fed or pastured sources, since that will make them lower in omega-6s and higher in omega-3s, but even then most contain a decent mix of the good mono and saturated fats. Bacon, for instance, is often said to be all saturated fat, but this is not the case; more than half of the fats in bacon are monounsaturated, which is the "healthy fat" that they talk about in avocados and olive oil!

Speaking of saturated fat, and its evil henchman, cholesterol, these two get blamed for arteriosclerosis and many other coronary ailments, but cholesterol and saturated fats are actually essential to our diets.

It is a common myth that eating cholesterol or saturated fat will raise your blood cholesterol. Many studies have shown that eating more or less cholesterol and saturated fat does little or nothing to increase or decrease the levels in your blood. Eat more and your body makes less, and eat less, and your body is forced to make more for itself. For the most part, blood cholesterol is self-limiting.

Again, concentrate on limiting the bad fats and increasing the fat (omega-3s) that really needs the boost and the rest tends to work itself out for the most part.

Good fats gone bad

A good, boring lecture on good and bad fats would not be complete without at least a cursory mention of what can make a good fat bad. Time, heat, and light.

Have you ever opened up a really old jar of peanut butter? Maybe a bottle of olive oil that you found in the back of the cupboard over the oven? It still looks tasty, but smells horribly stale. It's rancid. It doesn't have the obvious curdle of old milk or the rotting stench and mold of old meat, but it's bad, nevertheless. Don't use it. Time, heat, and light have destroyed it. Luckily the smell and taste are warnings to not use it.

Keep your oils fresh by buying what you will use in a reasonable time frame and keeping them cool and out of bright light. If you like, you can keep it in the refrigerator, which will keep it fresh longer. Some of the better oils come in opaque or dark green or brown glass, which helps to protect the oil at home and when it's still on the store shelves.

Cooking and overheating can also be a bad thing for many oils and fats. For cooking, choose oils with a high smoke point rather than low. Peanut oil is high (450°F), and is often used in stir frying for this reason. Coconut oil is becoming increasingly popular because of its many health benefits - you can get the expeller pressed version which is tasteless. Extra Light Olive Oil is a decent choice, too. While butter smokes at a low temperature, clarified butter has a much higher smoke point. Personally, when I do my high heat cooking, I choose coconut oil or clarified butter, which you can often buy as "ghee" in an Indian market.

Below, you will find a partial list of fats and oils, followed by their smoke points. Keep in mind that smoke point isn't everything; oils can still be bad for you (soybean, for instance), even when they have higher smoke points. ...they just don't smoke as easily. Also, a lower smoke point doesn't make them bad to cook with, just don't go with high heat.

The chart below starts with the highest smoke points, and goes down. For clarity, I have **bolded** some of the best choices for higher heat cooking, and left off the oils that I simply can't recommend (shortening, soybean oil, etc.). This is an abridged list, listing only common fats and oils. For a more complete list of fats and oils (both good and bad) see Appendix 3.

Healthy fats and their smoke points

Avocado oil – 520°F, 271°C

Clarified butter/Ghee – 485°F, 252°C

Canola oil (high oleic) – 475°F, 246°C

Olive oil (extra light) – 468°F, 242°C

Palm oil – 455°F, 235°C

Coconut oil (refined) – 450°F, 232°C

70

Peanut oil (refined) – 450°F, 232°C

Canola oil (refined) – 400°F, 204°C

Olive oil (virgin) – 391°F, 199°C

Canola oil (expeller pressed) – 375°F, 190°C

Olive oil (extra virgin) – 375°F, 191°C

Lard – 370°F, 188°C

Coconut oil (extra virgin) – 350°F, 177°C

Butter – 250–300°F, 121–149°C

As you can see by the butter vs. ghee (clarified butter) comparison, it's often the purity of the fat that makes or breaks a smoke point. Extra Virgin is tasty, but the tastiness is in the particles of olive that are left in the oil. On the other hand, Extra Light Olive Oil is rather tasteless, but a better choice for cooking. Extra Light Olive Oil has a smoke point of 468°F, which is good, while Extra Virgin Olive Oil has a pretty low smoke point of 375°F. Both are healthy, but use one for cooking and one for places where you are looking for good taste, like dressings. There are some oils that should never be used for cooking, like flaxseed and fish oil (yuck).

The "lard is bad for you" myth

1 – pork fat is 45% monounsaturated fat, which is the same fat that makes peanut oil a healthy choice.

2 – saturated fat (39% for lard) is necessary for hormone production and the rebuilding of healthy tissues throughout the body. Mother's milk, for instance is 54% saturated fat.

3 – since the dramatic decline in butter and lard consumption, heart disease has risen even faster.

3. Veggies

Our third tenet of a healthy diet is vegetables, an important source of nutrition. While different diet authors will argue what is or isn't a veggie, the fact is that most of us don't eat enough vegetables, period. We can argue whether a tomato, squash, or potato should count as a vegetable, but if you're not even eating those, you're already missing out on many valuable nutrients. Many vitamins and minerals, and phytonutrients, plus fiber, are found in vegetables, and there are very few diets that don't encourage more veggies. Even the Atkins Diet encourages veggies; it's after two weeks of an "induction period." Yeah, many people are surprised to hear that, but it's also true that many people apparently haven't actually read the Atkins Diet.

For the most part, vegetables are low calorie and pretty filling. Even higher calorie choices, like sweet potatoes, are fairly low in calories when not covered with marshmallows and butter, and since they contain fiber, they tend to help fill you up and keep you there.

4. Protein

Protein is the keystone to the success of your diet. Animal protein such as eggs, meat, fish, dairy, is a central part to a man's weight loss diet - it will keep you full, help you burn calories, help recover from workouts, and strengthen your immune system. Protein is how your body builds tissue, which is why it's so popular to grab a protein shake or bar after a workout.

You can get protein from plants, too, but it's harder to get all that you need without carefully balancing out your diet to include the more protein rich plant foods. Shoot for variety, you can have eggs at one meal, steak at another, chili or stir fry for dinner.

Protein helps us build sought after muscle and even keep muscle that we have when we are dieting. Protein makes us feel full quickly and keeps us feeling full until the next meal. Protein has been proven to help people stick to their diet plans longer, and the diets with the most protein usually result in the most weight loss. Who wouldn't like that?

5. Fruits

When eaten as part of a balanced diet, they contribute positively to your overall health. Like vegetables, fruits have plenty to write home about. They contain lots of vitamins, minerals, phytonutrients, and fiber, and relatively few calories for what you get out of them. There are low calorie fruits (berries) and high calorie fruits (bananas), but eating fruit tends to contribute positively to your overall health. I encourage you to choose fruits as snacks over processed, sugary desserts!

In the last few years, there's been plenty of controversy surrounding the innocent fruit. One group says "no one ever got fat from eating fruit," while the other camp claims that fruit has too much sugar, in general, or too much fructose specifically. Each side has a few valid arguments, but for most of us, the truth lies somewhere in between.

In general, I think fruit is a good part of a fat loss diet, and unless you are eating too much of it, including fruit in your diet is a good way to go.

6. Activity

A reasonable activity level is important to make your diet a success and keep you healthy. Although it's not really part of "diet," we're still making it an important part of our "Healthy diet tenets." Without a decent activity level, you will never be as healthy as you could be. I firmly believe that you need activity to be healthy. You don't need to run marathons or be an Olympic lifter, but you need to do more than watch sports and think about hiking, you need to actually get up and get out there.

The popular saying "you can't outrun bad nutrition" is a pretty accurate slogan for most people. For the most part, the guys who spout off that quote are saying that you'll never get as lean or as healthy as you want while you're still eating a lot of crap. It's mostly true, as it's pretty hard to cardio off the 900 extra calories in those donuts this morning. You just can't run off 900 extra calories every time you overeat and expect to lose the fat you want. Really, only high level athletes can "run" fast enough or far enough to escape those extra calories. Even then, what happens when the athlete stops running?

Even though you can't really outrun bad nutrition, exercise can still do a lot to help. Exercise, and the type of exercise, helps to determine where extra calories go when you eat more than you need, and what you burn off when you eat less than you need. Also, an active lifestyle can actually go a long way to improve the health markers that you would think only come from being slim; high blood pressure and bad cholesterol readings, joint pain, blood sugar issues, low libido and depression can all be improved by taking up a more active lifestyle. Still, as many pro-obesity web sites and groups are fond of pointing out, you can be pretty "healthy" and still be overweight, so exercising or not, you have to watch your diet for best results.

We're not suggesting that you eat what you want and just train to make up for it – you'll still be fat, after all. You don't want that, do you?

The "healthy diet tenets," one more time

Remember, we're talking about what makes a diet healthy or not healthy, and the evidence seems to point out that sensible calories, the right fats, the right amount of protein, the inclusion of vegetables and fruits, and a decent activity level are what it's going to take to make a diet healthy.

> 1. **Calories** – only as many as you need
>
> 2. **Fats** – avoid the bad and look for the good
>
> 3. **Veggies** – vegetables are full of fiber and nutrients… eat up!
>
> 4. **Protein** – muscle building and filling
>
> 5. **Fruits** – it's what's for dessert
>
> 6. **Activity** – either hunt and gather for the first 5 tenets or head outside to play

Reading the label

I just talked about all of the components that make up a healthy lifestyle, including things like protein, fats, and calories. I also talked about the importance of looking out for the "good guys" and the "bad guys," but where do you look for these things?

Most of the foods that you make yourself won't actually have ingredients, but are ingredients in and of themselves; meat, vegetables, milk, coconut oil, butter, etc. These things should be relatively simple to understand. They may have some ingredients other than the thing that they are, but the list of components should be short and sweet. Packaged foods, on the other hand, might contain ingredients so long that they have to print them so small that you need a microscope to read them all. Let's talk about how to read these lists and make smart decisions about the foods that you are considering buying and eating.

Nutrition Facts

When picking up packaged foods it's important to take a look at the nutrition label, labeled "Nutrition Facts," on the back. It gives you all the information you need to make a good choice about whether to buy it, eat it, or serve it.

Nutrition Facts

Serving Size (30g)
Servings Per Container 3.5

Amount Per Serving

Calories 140 — Calories from Fat 25

%**Daily Value***

Total Fat 3g	**5%**
Saturated Fat 1g	**5%**
Trans Fat 0.5g	
Polyunsaturated Fat 1.5g	
Monounsaturated Fat 0.5g	
Cholesterol 30mg	**10%**
Sodium 55mg	**2%**
Total Carbohydrate 25g	**8%**
Dietary Fiber 1g	**4%**
Sugars 9g	
Sugar Alcohol 0g	
Protein 3g	

Vitamin A 4%   •   Vitamin C 0%

Calcium 8%   •   Iron 0%

* Percent Daily Values are based on a 2,000 calorie diet. Your Daily Values may be higher or lower depending on your calorie needs:

	Calories:	2,000	2,500
Total Fat	Less than	65g	80g
Sat Fat	Less than	20g	25g
Cholesterol	Less than	300mg	300mg
Sodium	Less than	2,400mg	2,400mg
Total Carb		300g	375g
Dietary Fiber		25g	30g

Servings and servings per container

If you skip directly down to the second line, you should see "servings per container." This can be an eye opener, right there. Logically, you'd think that a snack size package, for instance, would contain a snack, but you'll often find that there could be 2, 3 or 4 servings even in a tiny little package!

Even more mysteriously, you'll often find *fractional* servings. A package of gas station peanuts should contain one serving of nuts, but over the last couple of years, competition between peanut "manufacturers" has inflated the contents of those little bags to 1.75 (even 1.9) servings. A serving is usually 150 calories, and now you are faced with a package containing 263 calories and more. Sure, you can stop after one serving, but who does that?

Calories

As you can see in the fine print just above the word calories, this is *per serving*. Just make sure that you multiply the calories by the amount of servings you intend to eat.

I absolutely love a certain company's protein cookies. Those delicious soft cookies come in a single package of two. The package is folded in a way that you see the nutrition info in a way that makes you think it's per package, when it's actually per cookie. You might think that the whole package is only 200 calories, but if you eat both cookies you will be consuming 400 calories. Just try to stop at one – these are to die for...

Galya recently found a big cookie at a cafe, and because it's one cookie, it's likely meant to be a snack for just one person. But, after reading the label, she saw the cookie was 3.5 servings and 525 calories of true calorie bomb! She couldn't find two and a half friends to share the cookie, so she put it back...

The serving size and the calories per serving are the two most important things on the nutrition label, since ultimately your calorie intake will determine your progress far more than how many grams of fat, carbs, protein or fiber the food contains.

Calorie bomb, noun

> *1 – any food that contains a ridiculous amount of calories*

> *2 –a meal that's large and bad enough to ruin all dieting progress for the past week*

> *3 – one of those huge burritos that are only made in America*

Fat

Ideally, a healthy diet should contain mostly natural fats, equally distributed between saturated, monounsaturated and polyunsaturated fats. Don't worry if a food only has saturated or monounsaturated fat, since other foods throughout the day contain the other fats. Your cheese might be mostly saturated fat, but the olive oil in salad will mostly contain monounsaturated fats. The most important thing to know about fat is to make sure there are no trans-fats or hydrogenated fats on the label. These fats are very detrimental to your cardiovascular and metabolic health.

Cholesterol

Cholesterol has a bad reputation because of a number of misread and misused studies from a long time ago. Now we know that cholesterol in food has little to do with your risks of high cholesterol and cardiovascular disease. In fact, certain foods, such as eggs, that are high in cholesterol, may actually improve your cholesterol profile. Your body has a way of self-regulating and for the most part will make less cholesterol to offset the amount of cholesterol that you eat. Cholesterol is used by your body for cell structures, as well as the production of hormones, such as testosterone. Shooting for a diet low in cholesterol isn't always the best choice.

Sodium

It's salt, and other taste enhancers. In packaged foods, you often find more sodium than in the varieties of the same food you would prepare yourself. Also, the sodium number on the label includes sodium found in the controversial ingredient known as MSG (monosodium glutamate). If you are monitoring the sodium in your diet, this is an important number to watch out for. If you are particularly concerned about MSG, you have to go down to the ingredient label to scan for that particular type of sodium.

Carbohydrates

Carbohydrates are both tolerated and condemned by different nutrition camps. The truth is that different bodies can tolerate wide ranges and varying levels of carbohydrate. From a nutritional standpoint, your body can live almost entirely without carbohydrates. One organ in your body that most critically needs carbohydrate is your brain, but if pressed, the liver can actually produce all that you need.

It's not always the amount of the carbohydrates that's the issue, but the calories that come from the carbohydrates, since they can be quickly and disastrously overeaten. We are naturally drawn to the taste of foods that are sweet, and combined with the ease of chewing, swallowing, and digesting of processed foods and sugary drinks – it's no wonder that we often overeat them.

Carbohydrates from natural sources, such as fruits, vegetables, grains and dairy are also better tolerated than the carbs you tend to find in a milk shake or a can of soda. The total carbohydrate listed isn't all that important, but if you see that a large percentage of the calories in that food is coming from carbs and sugars, make sure that you eat something else at that meal, such as protein or fat, to slow down the absorption of the carbohydrate, since foods high in that macro tend to cause rapid increase in energy and then the sudden drops that encourage hunger and the urge to overeat. In nature, it takes a large amount of food to get a high amount of carbs, but this is not the case with packaged, processed foods, and sweetened beverages.

Fiber

After you read many nutrition labels, you'll start to notice that the more natural the food is, the more fiber it will tend to have relative to its total carb content. A higher fiber content usually means that the carb sources in the foods are less processed and closer to their natural form. Whole wheat, for instance, still contains the husk and bran that's been removed from the white flour used to make most bread, cookies, and tortillas. The husk and bran are what contain most of the fiber in the grain, not to mention most of the vital micro-nutrients. You won't see most of these micro-nutrients listed on a nutrition label, but seeing a high fiber number is one clue that they are still there. Not all foods will have high fiber content, but when you see a high carb food with little to no fiber, that should be a warning to look deeper and reconsider this food.

Protein

The front labels of many processed foods focus on fat and carbs, and it's common to see "low carb" or "fat free!" splashed across a box of snacks. It's fairly uncommon to see any mention of the protein, and when it does, it's often highlighting a "high" protein content of 10 or even 5 grams of protein! Sure, a snack bar containing 10g of protein might be pretty high compared to a Pop Tart, but that doesn't mean it's high, good, or good for you.

For the most part, protein has been a neglected area of mainstream diets, but protein is pretty important for a number of reasons. Protein helps build and maintain muscle and keeps your metabolism high so that you can burn more fat. Most importantly, a diet higher in protein gets you full faster and keeps you feeling full longer. Studies have shown that people lose more weight on diets higher in protein.

When reading a nutrition label, keep in mind that not all proteins are created equal. There are proteins that come from animals and plants, and in general, animal proteins are more easily used by your body. Vegetable proteins contain lower amounts of protein compared to their carbohydrate and fat percentages, so in order to get a significant amount of protein from plants, you might need to eat more calories than you would with animal sources.

Ingredients

In addition to the macro-nutrients (fat, protein, fiber, etc.), the nutrition label contains a list of all the ingredients that are in that food. You can never tell exactly how much of a food is in the item, but they are listed by volume. The more of each item in the food, the higher on the list it appears.

Too long, did not eat

If the ingredient list for a food is too long, it's unlikely that you will read the whole thing, but you might still eat it. That's probably a mistake.

While it is technically possible to have a really long list of ingredients and still be a healthy and a high quality food, the odds are not good. A very long list of ingredients is almost assuredly a sign of a highly processed product. If it's too long, it's not usually worth reading, much less eating.

Good Guys & Bad Guys

There are those who say there are no bad foods. Others believe it's the addition of specific foods or supplements that's the key to health. I believe it's a bit of both. There certainly are bad foods out there (trans-fats, for example), and no amount of fish oil or vitamins pills can make up for those.

Instead of looking for the magic pill to good health and fat loss, use our lists of good guys and bad guys to maximize the good and minimize the bad. As with most things, perfection is not the goal. The goal is finding a good balance between leading a happy life and having a healthy body.

The good guys

There are foods that nature intended for us, and therefore help us maintain optimal weight and health, and help us to feel happy, productive, and energized. Try to make these "good guy" foods 90% of your nutrition:

Focus on these good guys

water

butter

ghee (clarified butter)

olive oil

avocado

nuts in shell

coconut and coconut oil

meat

poultry

fish and shellfish

whole eggs

milk

yogurt

cheese

cottage cheese

vegetables

root vegetables

fruits

potatoes and sweet potatoes

beans and legumes

unprocessed grains (limit)

fermented vegetables (kimchee, sauerkraut)

fermented/cultured drinks (kefir, kombucha, etc.)

The ~~really~~ bad guys

There are ingredients in our foods that prevent us from being at our optimal health, weight, and performance levels. You may see these as ingredients on boxes and labels, items on restaurant menus, or you may encounter them as actual foods in the grocery store. Either way, beware these foods. Avoid the following "bad guy" foods as best you can. These foods are no good!

Avoid these bad guys

Margarine, shortening, imitation and simulated butters

Trans fats, hydrogenated fats

Non-dairy creamers

High sodium foods

MSG (monosodium glutamate)

Corn oil, soybean oil, vegetable oil, and seed oils (sunflower, safflower, cottonseed, etc.)

The not quite as bad, but still bad, bad guys

There are also "bad guys" that are not optimal for health, but when consumed in small amounts and infrequently, they shouldn't ruin your health. The key is to keep them a small percentage of your diet, and an infrequent guest on your plate.

You want to keep these "bad guy" foods a small part of your diet; special occasions, a 10% meal, etc.

Minimize these bad guys

Sugar and sweets, high fructose corn syrup, agave syrup, things that make something sweet, no matter how "natural" they sound

Artificial sweeteners

Sodas and juices

Fancy coffee drinks

Alcohol

Heavily processed packaged foods

Deep fried/breaded foods

Bottled salad dressings and dressing mixes (often contain bad oils from the above list)

Soy products, with the exception of soy sauce, miso, tempeh, and other fermented soy products

Sesame oil (as a seed oil, it's "bad," but it's so flavorful that you don't use much. Enjoy it as a taste ingredient, but not as a cooking oil.)

Processed grains

Artificial colors and flavorings

Chemicals, preservatives, and things that you can't identify, recognize, and pronounce

E ingredients – "E" ingredients are the European system for listing artificial ingredients, colors, preservatives, and flavorings. They are listed as a capital E and three numerals (E621, E951 etc.). Not all Es are bad (paprika?), but a lot of Es is a bad sign.

Why go healthy, when you can just go for the fast fat loss?

Yes, you can lose weight – as the infamous Twinkie dieter of 2010 showed us – eating nothing but unhealthy foods. And, because of calorie restriction, you can even temporarily improve blood markers. So, if we can eat anything we want, and still lose weight, why would we even waste our time with eating healthier?

• Better satiety – healthier foods tend to be more filling and satisfying after they are eaten.

• Long term weight control – eating a diet of Twinkies teaches you nothing about living in the real world; you can't eat Twinkies forever.

• Long term health – your blood work is only better when you are eating less than you need to maintain your weight. As soon as you start to eat more again, you will suffer the consequences of a diet filled with empty calories, artificially delicious, and packed with the inflammatory agents of modern lifestyle diseases.

• Less inflammation – processed foods are packed with the "bad guys," which are filled full of anti-nutrients, inflammatory oils, plus sugary, low quality carbs. These can wreak havoc on your metabolism and health.

• Motivation – long term, dieting to lose weight loses its appeal. You can only be so hungry, and then you give up, telling yourself you'll be back at it tomorrow. Sometimes tomorrow never comes. But, when you eat right because you believe it's the better thing to do, you're much more likely to get back on the path when you do step off, and you'll stray less often.

• You just feel better – When you feel good, you move more, and when you move more, you burn more calories, work and play harder, and even rest and sleep better.

What about condiments?

Feel free to use iodized salt, Himalayan salt, sea salt, Morton's salt, plus all the herbs and spices you like. As for prepared condiments, dressings, and toppings, read all ingredient labels carefully, as they often contain sugar and many of the "bad guys" listed above. Moderation is the key.

Our clients often ask how strict they need to be with the good guys and bad guys, and it always depends on the client and the goal. But, as with most things, perfection is not the goal. The goal is finding a good balance between leading a happy life and having a healthy body.

Out with the bad, more room for the good

Our "healthy diet tenets" cover the important roles that calories, fats, vegetables, protein, fruits, and activity play in a healthy diet and lifestyle. You now know how to read a nutrition label, and what ingredients to avoid when you find them.

Seeing how our healthy diet tenets relate to modern diet & health phenomenon might also help you see how vegans, paleo dieters, vegetarians, low carbers, and peddlers of superfoods, fruit juices, and supplements can all find data that says that *they alone* hold the secret to good health! We can argue which diet is healthier than the others, but in this book we're concerned about diets that are healthy, period.

I'm sure you can see how most diets that are promoted as healthy and sustainable seem to have a lot in common, from eating less processed food, less sugar, more whole foods and vegetables, and hence, fewer calories. It's not necessary to choose an extreme diet to get healthy and fit, nor is it critical to choose *exactly* the right diet in order to succeed. The best diet for you is one that's healthy and flexible, so that you can stay motivated and stay on your plan.

Success in the spotlight #2

A teenager who lost the fat and kept it off

Kevin has been a friend of ours for many years. I have a special affinity for Kevin, because he also grew up less than lean, just like me.

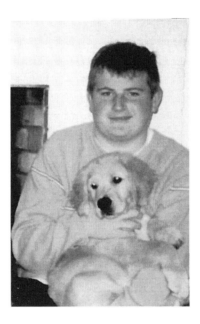

Unlike me, though, Kevin found the motivation early on, and as a young adult dropped the weight and got into shape.

In addition to finding his way to get and stay lean, Kevin found his passion in fitness and training; he created and hosts the best fitness podcast in the world, The FitCast, and now is a great trainer and strength coach in his own right!

Kevin Larabee, 26 years old, 195 lbs, 6 feet tall, and 35 lbs lighter

Galya – How old were you when you started losing weight?

Kevin – I was 15-16 years old, it was before I got my driver's license. Then my new body helped me get a girl in drivers Ed.

When I started, I dropped 35 lbs in 3 months.

Galya – What was wrong with your diet?

Kevin – Emotional eating after school. I was a big kid and got picked on. I wanted to be better at basketball. I wanted to be great at it. I was always a chubby kid. My parents were very strict with what I ate. After my parents got divorced they got more relaxed and used food to make me happier, so they cut me some slack.

Galya – What did you do to lose the weight?

Kevin – I was super active. I ate fruit and rice cakes. I decided to eat what I considered "healthy" foods. A year later I bought Testosterone Advantage Plan. I ate veggies with my family and I stayed away from the bad foods. I was working 40 hours a week at a grocery store. I kept myself busy. My parents got me a gym membership for my birthday in January. I remember eating lots of watermelon and sandwiches. I had no problem giving up my food. I had all the energy in the world.

Galya – Did your friends and relatives support you?

Kevin – I made my own food, mostly, but my parents bought the ingredients at the store. There were some subtle attempts at sabotage, like them offering to pick up some pizza for me, but they also got me a gym membership.

Galya – What about when you have to spend a long time with relatives, what are your strategies for meals?

Kevin – I tell them that I am training for something specific. I try to look busy with moving around amongst the friends and relatives. If I did know I was going to an event without great food options I would get in a hard training session with some sled work or sprints.

Galya – What in your opinion stops people from losing weight?

Kevin – I think people are reluctant to give up guy foods, like beer, real burgers and pizza. Sports and men go together, and not without food. If there were more healthy, but manly Super Bowl foods, that would be a huge thing for men.

Galya – How much weight have you lost over these years?

Kevin – 30 lbs altogether.

Galya – Had you ever tried to lose weight before you succeeded?

Kevin – I vaguely remember buying diet pills off Ebay.com. I would bring them to school and try to take them. I was worried it wouldn't be healthy. Any attempt at doing it was halfhearted.

Galya – If you could go back what would you have done differently?

Kevin – I would do weight training instead of running my ass off (literally). I would eat moderate protein and not low fat. Fruit is very important, too.

Galya – Which are your favorite books on fat loss and training?

Kevin – My favorite training books are The New Rules of Lifting by Alwyn Cosgrove and Lou Schuler and Maximum Strength by Eric Cressey. My favorite nutrition books are Leigh Peele's Fat Loss Troubleshoot and John Berardi's Precision Nutrition.

Galya – What are you doing now to maintain your weight?

Kevin – Fitness is my career now. I train clients and I am the host of TheFitCast Podcast. I think of my own fitness and nutrition as a part of my job. It's all about educating and keeping clients and motivating them.

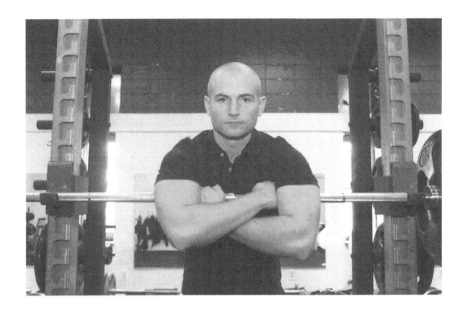

Kevin is currently an NSCA Certified Strength & Conditioning Specialist at Mike Boyle Strength & Conditioning, and the host of the extremely popular, long running, hilarious, and incredibly educational podcast known as TheFitCast (*thefitcast.com* and on iTunes).

In addition to his life as a coach and trainer, Kevin is an avid gamer, writer, and audio and video producer, yet he remains strong and lean; Kevin shows us all that a modern life isn't an obesity sentence, as long as you take care to eat right and get plenty of smart training and exercise.

7

Do I have to change who I am?

Early on, I told you that you were only going to change what you needed to change, and only when you needed to change it.

So far, you've learned a lot about nutrition, diet, and exercise. What a calorie means, macros, etc. We've shown you our Tenets of Healthy Eating, given you examples of how some people get fat, and how others stay slim. You've made some goals, you've been writing things down, and you've been exercising. Now is the time to make your first conscious change since you started reading this book.

Before you jump into this thing too deeply, too quickly, I want to give one little warning and one little reminder. The warning is "Don't do too much, too soon." The reminder is "This is a long term transformation, not a short term change."

Hopefully, you've already seen and felt some good stuff happening. You are energized and excited by the positive changes that you've felt over the past two weeks, so it's natural to want to hurry up and get things moving even faster. You might feel like taking up jogging and putting yourself on a Spartan-esque diet of nothing but chicken breasts and broccoli. Don't do it! You feel good now because it's early in the process and you've seen some good progress, but remember that you haven't yet had to make any big changes! Things aren't all that tough. That positive feeling might not be there in another two weeks if you make life too restrictive for yourself.

What if you're still waiting for things to change? You've been diligently writing down everything you eat and all of your activities. You started the Kickstart exercise program, but other than being a little sore, you've seen no real changes yet. Anxious to see some big changes, you start reading the upcoming list and make plans to implement them all, starting NOW!

Don't do it! I know you want results now, but don't you also want to succeed? Isn't your long term success more important than a short term loss that might easily be followed by gaining it all back? Extreme and restrictive diets like HCG or those lemon juice and pepper cleanses do seem to work for a while, but I don't know a single person who hasn't gained it all back or more, learned nothing in the process, and gotten more and more discouraged. Repeated failures in the fat loss department make it that much harder to even try again.

Too much, too soon, and you're likely to feel like you've been thrown into dieting prison, where you've lost all freedom and all control. At first, you'll feel some changes, and sticking it out won't seem so bad, but when things slow, and they will, you'll be frustrated, weak, and hungry. ...and quitting will be all too easy.

A long term transformation takes time. Yes, you can make the decision to transform *now*, but it's small changes, over time, that will get you to your goal. Remember, if you quit or backslide, you'll have to "transform" all over again. To increase the odds, increase the time. As long as you are seeing the progress that you need to move forward, resist making more and more changes that make things more and more restrictive.

More changes, right now, may seem good because they seem like they would get you to your goal even faster, but going fast, then getting discouraged and quitting is actually less good than finishing in the longer run, right?

Only change what you need to change, and only when you need to change it.

That's the goal oriented, change vs. transformation aspect. I haven't even talked about the realities of fat loss and time, and it involves a concept called "homeostasis."

The more things change, the more they stay the same

Or, more accurately, "the more *quickly* things change, the quicker your body will adapt." This is a good reason not to change things before you have to. This phenomenon is called homeostasis. In a nutshell, homeostasis is your body's charming ability, or annoying propensity, to adjust so that you "stay the same."

Have you dieted before and hit a plateau, staying the same weight for weeks or even months at a time? This is your body, trying very hard to stop losing weight. The underlying science, physics, and chemistry might be complicated, but the simple explanation is that your body wants to survive, and the way it does that is to keep all the muscle and fat it can for energy. Yep, your body thinks you are starving, so your metabolism is subconsciously slowed to stop any weight loss. Yay for survival!

As awesome as it is to know your chances for survival are good, it sucks that you've stopped losing weight. You're in this to lose fat, so something must be done to push beyond this little trick your body is pulling on you.

Every time your body self-adjusts to your lower calories or higher activity level, you have to take measures to sidestep its plan to stop the losses. This may be lowering calories further, stepping up your activities, cutting carbohydrates, or changing your exercise plan to a tougher one. If you do all of this *now*, before you have to, your body will still adjust to those levels, but where will you go from here? You've already done so much, early on, that you don't have a lot of new tricks to pull.

Understand that your body does its best to self-adjust as quickly as possible, and it will, whether you've set yourself up for slow and steady fat loss or fast and dramatic losses. Soon enough, your body will hit that plateau, and you have to have a next trick ready to go, so don't waste them all now! Enjoy the ride, and be ready to change paths. Be ready...

Low hanging fruit

You know now *not* to pull out all the stops on day one, but to save your moves for when you next need them. But, how do you know what to do next? Do you run harder, walk more, add more protein, count calories, and eat less fruit? It might be any one of those, but it is definitely the "low hanging fruit" that you reach for!

Low hanging fruit, noun

1 – the fruit that grows low on a tree and is therefore easy to reach

2 –a course of action that can be undertaken quickly and easily as part of a wider range of changes or solutions to a problem: first pick the low hanging fruit

---

As you can see by the dictionary definition, above, the analogy of picking the low hanging fruit is perfect for telling us how to select our "next step" toward further fat loss. In the very first pages of this book, I promised you that you'd only change what you had to change, when you had to change it. This is easier on you, of course, which both eases you into things, but also makes it less disruptive on your life. In this case, picking the low hanging fruit means taking the next step that's easiest on you, the least disruptive, and is just effective enough to keep weight loss progressing steadily OR kickstart further fat loss when you do hit a plateau.

What to change and when to change it

So, it's about two weeks since you started the "Kickstart," and you're wondering what, if anything, to do next.

You will use the charts that follow to determine your next move in training or nutrition, starting from the simplest and easiest, to the tougher and more complicated methods.

Follow the steps below, starting at the top, and only continue down to the next step when you're no longer seeing any progress. If you use up all your moves now, what will you do when you really need one?

This section shows you the steps you will be taking toward achieving your final goal – whether it's losing 5, 25, 50 lbs, or even more.

You might achieve your goals before reaching the bottom of the list, or at virtually any point along the way, so start reading, but only do something new when you really need it!

It's not a race. Baby steps…

Make sure to take at least two weeks to settle in to each step before adding in the next one. However, if after two full weeks, you haven't noticed a positive change, it's time to move on to the next step and make a change.

• Implement the latest step in your nutrition and/or training, then allow yourself two weeks to see whether it's working or not.

• If you notice positive changes as a result of your latest changes, then continue on without making any new changes. You don't really need to change much, if anything, if all is going well. Remember that too much change, too quickly can lead to trouble, both in motivation and in progress itself.

Remember how we talked about homeostasis and the body's ability to adjust to anything you throw at it? You need to keep some tricks in the bag, ready to pull out, just for when your body pulls this homeostasis *crap* on you!

• If, after two weeks of following instructions and trying your best, you still haven't noticed positive change, you're going to consider a next step. This is not a bad thing, as we're constantly fighting our own body's desire to stay the same. Take a final look at that last step to make sure you did things right, then move down to the next one. It's time to make another change.

• If, after those two weeks, you are still making steady progress, you don't need to do anything new. If you like, feel free to make small tweaks to your diet and exercise routines, but you don't need to do anything drastic. Many people like to merely fine tune their diet at this point, going healthier still or just naturally finding that they no longer need that late night snack. It's common to feel empowered by your progress, and find that you want to improve some on a regular basis. Enjoy that feeling and continue to improve, just don't make major changes unless they are necessary. Keep something in the bag…

Plateau Busters

Weight or waist hasn't budged in a loooong time? Did anything else happen recently that might have compromised your progress with your latest changes? Did you stop or slow down on exercising? Did you go off the diet too many times? Were you injured, depressed, or sick? Overworked and overtired?

Rather than panic and dramatically drop the calories or start running even farther, try these first:

• *Do you rely on artificial sweeteners? Try dropping them ALL for 30 days.*

• *Meditate, yoga, vacation, massage, foam roll, etc. Find a way to reduce stress.*

• *Have you been training forever? Consider a training break.*

• *Get more sleep and rest.*

• *Train less, walk more.*

Remember, that if you experience a stall, but you know you could have done better, it's probably time to knuckle down and give it *more time*. Before you add in another restriction or activity that might further frustrate you, try again for another two weeks, and give it your best shot!

If you truly feel that you've done it all right, but there has still been no progress, then it's time to take the next step on the list. Just one more step, though. They build on each other to bring you closer to your goal while avoiding drastic changes and restrictions *and* hopefully allowing you to continue to have some fun and enjoy the process.

Now, let's take a look at the steps and get started. They are divided into two categories; one for your diet and nutrition, and one for your training, activity, and exercise.

The nutrition steps

Step 1: The Kickstart Nutrition

Unless you're reading this book in one sitting, you should already be logging your food and taking your fish oil. You've probably already started this step – good job! Fish oil is important, because most of us need more of these valuable omega-3 fats. In addition, logging your food will allow you to troubleshoot your diet and help with the next steps. Be sure to log your food for at least one week before moving onto the next step. Of course, if you're still making progress, just keep logging and popping fish oil.

Step 2: Avoid empty calories

In order to determine where they come from look over your logs and circle all sweet drinks, candy, sweets and treats, and grain containing or grain based snacks. Consider some healthy substitutes for snacks: string cheese, raw or roasted nuts, beef jerky, protein shakes, or a piece of fruit. If you really need to have sweet drinks, such as Coke, switch to diet and give unsweetened tea, green tea, and soda water a try.

Step 3: Become a calorie detective

This is the time to use your food log to look up common foods that you eat and become familiar with their calorie content. For example this is when you find that the Grande Wet Burrito has 1600 calories, and three tacos have 900 calories. This is where you find that a double cheeseburger with fries has 1200 calories, and two single cheeseburgers have 600 calories. This is where you find that mustard has zero calories, and mayonnaise has 60 calories per serving. You will naturally start to choose meals with fewer calories and find out that they are just as filling as their higher calorie cousins.

Step 4. Substitute vegetables for "carbs" in your meals

Look at your main meals: breakfast, lunch, dinner. Where can you skip the bread, potato or rice, and insert some vegetables in their place? At our house, we often have a large salad, followed by a nice piece of meat with a side of roasted vegetables, and another small salad.

It's very very filling and definitely makes you not miss the garlic bread and mashed potatoes. There are many veggies to choose from – from simple lettuce and steamed Brussels sprouts to slow roasted beets and spaghetti squash. The recipes in the cookbook section will give you plenty of ideas.

Bunless burgers and the side salad

My favorite burger joint, In-N-Out Burger, has no salad or vegetable options, but I still go. You see, a lettuce wrapped burger often has as many veggies as a burger and a side salad. I've bought them both and done the weighing and measuring for you. It's not really that the lettuce wrapped burgers have enough veggies, but it's more a reminder of how little nutrition is in one of those side salads.

Just to be safe, order extra tomatoes, pickles, onions, peppers, and whatever else passes for a veggie on that burger. You're still better off than the side salad because you don't waste calories on that unhealthy dressing.

As a plus for cheapskates, now you don't have to buy a side salad.

Step 5. Follow the Healthy Diet Tenets

Ensure that you are following the Healthy Diet Tenets that I outlined in the nutrition chapter. You may need to go over your log and see if you have opportunities to include more protein, healthy fats and vegetables, and you may need to refer to the hierarchy of training to remind yourself to optimize your daily activities and plan training sessions. Spend at least two weeks doing that until you go to the next step.

Step 6. Time your carbs

Remove non-veggie carbs from all non-post workout meals. That means you get to eat rice, potatoes, pasta or bread *only* after a training session or a long hike. This will pull much needed nutrients for recovery inside the muscle tissue, but it will leave a big portion of your day carbohydrate free so you can use your own fat for energy. The recipe section offers many ways to add vegetables to your meals, so you don't feel hungry or deprived. Do this for at least 2 weeks before you move on to the next step.

Step 7. Count calories

My advice is to start counting calories *only* when you are no longer seeing results from removing carbohydrate and otherwise making conscious efforts to simply eat better and eat less. With luck, and with your new understanding of how food and exercise work with the body, I hope it never comes to this, but if it does, it should be many weeks before you need to resort to this step. If things continued to go great, you may have achieved your fat loss goals without any calorie counting, and as a result, ended up on a sunny beach somewhere, showing off your hard earned "abs."

To count calories, you will need a rough idea of how much you are eating, so you will need to buy a food scale and start using a calorie calculator, such as Fitday.com, CalorieKing.com, Livestrong.com, or another online program that you can easily access from your computer. There are also many programs that you can use on your smartphones that will allow you to see how much you are eating.

Count your calories and track your body weight over the next few weeks. If your weight is stable then the calories you are eating are enough to maintain it. Calculate your weekly average so you can move on to Step 8.

Step 8. Reduce calories

You know your caloric level of maintenance from the previous step – now the only thing you need to do is to lower your intake by 10%. You can cut them a bit from every meal or cut them all from just one meal – it's really up to you. Some people skip a meal, such as their afternoon snack, others split their lunch in two and eat it for lunch and a small snack. Either way, you need to find a way to eat 10% fewer calories. You can research some of the many ways to cut calories, such as calorie cycling, intermittent fasting, etc. as they will all help you decrease calories while still enjoying a variety of foods.

If, after a week or two, you still don't see a drop on the scale, reduce calories by another 10% until you see progress.

The training steps

Step 1: The Kickstart Training Program

You've likely been doing the Kickstart Training Program for about two weeks now, doing it 2 times a week. At any point after starting the Kickstart, you can take a look at Step 2. If you're still making progress, feel free to continue.

Step 2: Start the Fat Loss Training Program

It's time to step up your training. Do the Fat Loss Routine up to 2 times a week. When you feel that you can do more move on to step 4. Remember, if you are making progress, you don't have to move to step 3 and 4 yet, but you may if you want to train more.

Like I talked about in the nutrition flowchart, always take 2 weeks to get comfortable with any changes before moving onto the next step.

Step 3: Find movement opportunities

Do the Life Questionnaire and identify ways to add more movement into your life wherever possible. Remember that you aren't looking to add a weekly marathon or start riding a bike to work, but you do want to get up and move around more, whether it's more of the shopping, cleaning, playing with the kids, or walking the dog.

If you have a pedometer, start using it. Studies have shown that people who get about 10,000 steps a day tend to lose more weight than those who walk less. If your numbers are lower, see what you can do to increase your steps!

Fitbit – the pedometer on steroids

A pedometer counts your steps for you, giving you a good idea of your activity levels throughout the day, but we highly recommend you take it a step further and order a Fitbit. This tiny, electronic pedometer can ride in your pocket, so no one even sees it. When you're near your computer, it beams your steps to the Fitbit website so you can track steps over time. Fitbit.com has great online food and exercise tracking, too! One of the biggest benefits of the Fitbit is learning just how much we tend sit around and do nothing – time in the car, on the computer, and on the toilet reading books and newspapers adds up to tons of nothing.

Step 4: Add a workout

Start doing 3 workouts a week. In the meantime, pay attention to your other non-exercise activities that you tried to optimize in Step 2. Look at your steps – are you getting close to 10,000 steps a day? Did you buy, beg, borrow, or steal a pedometer yet? Finding out how much (or how little) you walk could go a long way to explaining the problem...

Step 5: Get more conditioned

When you are already doing your 3 workouts a week and you feel like you want to do extra activity, add 1 conditioning workout a week. Remember that too much training can ramp up your appetite and make your diet difficult. However, one session of very intensive conditioning training a week can really bump up the fat loss when you've hit a stall. Remember that it's important to ramp up exercise slowly, so make sure you give it two (or even four) weeks to see if your conditioning workouts are having the desired effect!

Step 6: Move more

Revise your non exercise movement (called NEAT or NEPA around the internet), and see if you can start logging 11,000-12,000 steps a day. Do this for two weeks.

NEAT stands for Non Exercise Activity Thermogenesis, while NEPA stands for Non Exercise Physical Activity. I know it's semantics, but no matter what someone types in an online forum, you can't do more NEAT, but you can do more NEPA, which can lead to more NEAT. Neat, huh?

Step 7: Condition red!

If you still have the drive and energy, feel free to add another conditioning session (but do not exceed three sessions) to your schedule, but we'd almost prefer if you walk more, put on a backpack with 20-25 lbs of weight in it, or take hikes. Lower intensity exercise, coupled with movements that are new to you, have added weight, or over uneven terrain, might burn more fat than extra sprints without the risk of making you extra hungry.

8

All about exercise

Training for fat loss

In the beginning of the book I gave you the Kickstart Program, where you immediately started doing *something* and stopped doing *nothing*. The Kickstart Program might have been a true introduction to training for some of you, and maybe just a reintroduction to others. We've all come from different backgrounds, from those of you who are former athletes, to people like me, who did little more than sit around.

In this chapter, you will learn why exercise is so important to losing weight and easily keeping it off. I also go over some common types of exercise and teach you how they fit in your life so you can choose the ones that give you the biggest bang for your buck.

"But wait, I am already training and I know what I am doing."

That's just fine, and I'm happy to hear it! To you, things might come easier, because you can rely on a program that you know is working well for you! Read on, and make sure you refer to our hierarchy of training chart to determine whether you are focusing on the right *type* of exercise for fat loss!

The benefits of exercise

There are tremendous health benefits to exercise, as you know. Exercise decreases your risk of cardiovascular disease, fends off diabetes, prolongs your life and helps you sleep better. It fights depression, improves your libido, heightens concentration, and helps you have better relationships and social lives.

Of course, exercise also helps you lose weight. It does that in two ways; first you burn calories while you exercise, so it encourages your body to pull extra energy from your body (your own body fat is stored energy, for instance).

Second, it increases the number of calories you burn at rest, even while you are merely recovering. That's right; you will expend more energy while just sitting there! In the hours and days after exercise, your body needs to use extra energy to build muscle, make bones and ligaments stronger, etc. This is called the recovery period, and it's when you might feel sore, fatigued, or even get that certain feeling in your lungs that reminds you that you worked out *hard* earlier!

Exercise takes your diet to the next level

We have seen that people who exercise adhere better to their diets. You train and you feel good so you are less likely to reach for a second serving of ice cream. When you train and you can feel your hardening abs under your skin, you look forward to one day showing them off, and you're less likely to drink that fourth beer.

Exercise also improves feelings of accomplishment and motivation so you are more likely to maintain a healthy eating lifestyle.

Exercise is also your secret weapon and super tool for cushioning a larger meal. You can train prior to a large Thanksgiving buffet and rest assured most of the calories will feed the muscle while you are still torching fat.

Best of all, exercise affects your hormones and causes most of the food energy you eat to be directed toward muscle tissue, organs and bones, so your fat cells have nothing left to store. That's right - you get more muscle and less fat. Win-win.

Nutritionist and exercise expert Dr. John Berardi tells us how our thoughts on exercise calories have changed over time. "First, we thought exercise 'worked' because of the calories burned DURING the exercise session itself. Next, we thought exercise 'worked' because of the calories burned AFTER the exercise session. Now, we're thinking that exercise 'works' by directing nutrient traffic. In other words, exercise impacts gene expression, hormonal release, and nutrient uptake. So it's less about the calories and more about nutrient traffic control."

But, can you still lose weight without all that exercise? Sure, and here's the truth; you don't NEED to exercise to lose fat. If you can achieve a caloric deficit through eating less than your body needs, you will lose fat. But remember back when I talked about body composition? Remember that not all weight is created equal? If you lose 10 lbs without exercising or 10 lbs with exercise, will you look and feel the same?

If you lose weight with no exercise, chances are you will lose muscle together with fat. This might end up decreasing your metabolism and your energy levels as you lose weight. Over time, despite the weight lost, this can equate to easier weight gain and harder weight loss. It can make weight loss harder in the long run and make you feel softer and flabbier.

When you make exercise a regular part of your life, you will lose fat – primarily fat – and have a body that you're proud to show off once the fat is gone. In addition, your hard earned muscle will protect you against easy fat gain in the future. You will be like Bryan (remember that jerk from earlier?) the guy who enjoys food, exercises a bit, and stays the same happy and handsome weight. The other option, where you don't exercise, will just have you fluctuating between a skinny-fat Chandler and a fat-fat Chandler, neither of which is a winning situation.

How much exercise do you really need to lose fat?

Most of the people we interviewed said they wish they were better informed about exercise when they first started losing weight. Now that they know *how little* they actually need, they realize that they could have spent less time jogging, swimming, or power walking, and more time planning their diets. They would have also had more time to have fun and more time spent with loved ones.

They also told us they wish they had known more about how food determined the rate at which you lose fat, and how exercise just helped them on their way. This is almost the *reverse* of the conventional wisdom. It's unfortunate, but true; exercise, without good nutrition, will do little to no good.

Maybe you think you need to exercise a lot, run every morning and lift weights after work five times per week, when in fact you need very little exercise for fat loss. You might need a lot to improve an athletic ability or to put on slabs of meat on a skinny frame, but for actual fat loss you need less exercise than you really thought, just exercise properly targeted.

I don't expect you to make exercise your number one priority, I just expect you to make it a part of your life, whether it's a short time every day, 4 days a week, two days a week, or just on your weekend, but I do want you to make it a lasting part of your life.

The hard learned truth is that too much exercise will just make you hungry, tired, and leave you feeling beat up. As physical therapist and fitness expert Bill Hartman says: "more isn't better, better is better!"

I want you to make the best use of exercise, so we'll tell you how to choose the type that will get you to your goals fast and let you maintain your results with the least effort.

What is the best exercise for fat loss?

Almost all exercise is good, but not all exercise is created equal. The most common exercise people start doing when they want to lose weight is running. But have you ever looked at a runner and thought something just doesn't look right?

Bill Hartman tells us "You get in shape to run; you don't run to get in shape." Running is a natural activity, but unfortunately the typical guy that needs to lose fat is too out of shape to run safely. A friend recently said "but our ancestors did it." Of course, but they did not sit on chairs all day from the age of six, did not sit on toilets, and did not drive cars. Your body is not your ancestral body. Ankles, knees, hips and shoulders are far from being in good alignment. Desk bound jobs change the way our muscles work and make running often unsafe. You can't just run, you need to run well.

Apply the above to any dynamic sport and you will see how picking up a random sport with the intent to lose fat may not be the best solution.

> *If you are out of shape and attempt to do a very vigorous activity or play a sport, the structures in your body may be too stressed out, even if you don't have pain. This low level stress may even drive your appetite sky high or simply not allow you to recover and make the expected progress in your fat loss!*

So what would you do if you can't run? Walk, or walk uphill. Walk fast, walk a lot. Or swim, or bike. Or use the elliptical trainer. Or join a group exercise class.

But why do you turn to long duration, aerobic exercise in the first place? Somehow, someway, you learned that this is the type of exercise that burns fat, but this is just a leap of faith. Aerobic exercise, as studied, was never the best way to fat loss. It is good as a way to improve cardiovascular health, and it does so. It also improves your tolerance to blood sugar and helps you fight stress and sleeping disorders. It's also a way to burn some extra calories without taxing the system too much. All that being said, it won't *necessarily* help you burn all that much more fat.

The myth of the "fat burning zone" and cardio

Yes, the myth.

There are two primary myths about low intensity cardio and fat burning. The first is that you need to exercise for at least 20 minutes before you start burning fat. The second is that you need to exercise with a heart rate of about 65% to optimize fat burning. With these things in place, they say, you are in the zone. The fat burning zone!

The bad news is that it's a myth. The good news is also that it's a myth. How about that?

The 20 minute myth – At any given time, your body is burning a mixture of glycogen (sugar) and triglycerides (fat), with varying percentages, depending on the type of activity and the duration. Run for half an hour and most of the energy you burn for the first 20 minutes will indeed be mostly glycogen, but as your sugar reserves drop, you will use more and more fat, but it's hardly like a switch got flipped. You always burn some fat and you always burn some sugar, but it's a constantly varying ratio.

The 65% of maximum heart rate myth – This one is similar, but different. This one says that you burn the most fat at 60-65% of your Max Heart Rate. Yeah? Maybe? These studies were actually using VO2 max, not Max Heart Rate AND it's by ratio again, just like the 20 Minute Myth. No matter the heart rate (or percent of VO2 max), you always burn some fat and some glycogen. No switches are flipped here, either.

These areas are where scientific fact was understood, but applied wrong, leading the entire fitness industry in the wrong direction for many, many years. In fact, virtually every cardio machine and heart rate monitor in production has a setting or sticker telling you how to stay in the fat burning zone. Embarrassing...

Low intensity aerobic exercise does burn a higher percentage of fat than other forms of exercise, but that doesn't mean anything to your results, since fat loss is a big picture, 24/7 process - fat burning is not an event confined to your exercise periods. At some point we thought the more fat we used during exercise, the better. This, of course, is forgetting how many calories we were burning over a longer period of time.

Our logic excluded the effect that the type of exercise has on metabolism during rest. You don't lose much fat during exercise, no matter what you do. You lose fat the rest of the time. If you have a 168 hour week and spend 7 hours of it running, do you think it's the fat you lost during the 7 hours or during the 161 hours that really mattered in the 3 lbs that you lost last week? What if you burn an ounce of fat in 30 minutes? That's 270 calories, right? What if you spent that half an hour burning 400 calories worth of glycogen? What does it matter where the calories come from?

If you eat and train into a caloric deficit, your body will replace the calories you are missing from the fat that you want to lose. The more calories you expend, the better. Whether they come from fat or glucose is irrelevant. For those of you nit pickers, it might be cool to know that to an extent it *does* matter, because if you exercise more intensely, you are more likely to burn more calories from fat at rest. Since aerobic exercise is lower intensity, it is *less* likely to improve your expenditure at rest.

Good news, bad news

This is one myth that brings with it both good and bad. Good because you can focus your energy on other things that are far more time efficient and beneficial, like strength training and conditioning. It's bad news because you can no longer rely on the low intensity cardio that was so damned easy...

Regarding aerobic exercise; you don't have to do it at all, but if you have the time to, certainly do it. Just do it after you've done enough of the more important types of exercise that I am about to cover.

Strength training, resistance exercise, or lifting weights

Strength training falls into a very special category. Remember, not all exercise is created equal, so some types are better than other types. Weight training as we know it today originated both as a way to rehabilitate injured soldiers and as a way to entertain bored circus goers. Only in recent years have we come to see the growing amount of research that supports weight training for non-aesthetic or athletic purposes. Because of its nature, it has dramatic metabolic and cardiovascular benefits. It expends a lot of calories during and after training and sends most of the calories we consume toward the active tissues. It so happens that the way we use weights forces our bodies to work mostly in the 30 second to one minute exercise zone, slowly depleting our storage of glycogen and heavily relying on a huge influx of energy for recovery in the post workout window.

Unlike aerobic training, it's really hard to adapt to weight training, as you slowly get stronger and increase the resistance or complexity of exercises as you go. Thus you keep burning more calories and building active, calorie consuming tissue (muscle) - something that just cardio won't do for you.

Weight training recruits a large percentage of the muscle cells, unlike aerobic training, and thus makes them active at rest. On top of all, it is easy to do, you don't need special clothes or elaborate expensive equipment, and you can do it in the comfort of your own home. For most of the people we interviewed for this project, it is the preferred form of exercise, since it saves a lot of time and improves overall well-being like no other exercise they've tried.

Just like with all exercise, you have to bear in mind that if you end up compensating for your exercise efforts with extra food, even though some of it will be spent for muscle recovery, you will not be able to lose fat. Fat loss happens through caloric deficit, either caused by eating less, greater energy expenditure, or a combination of eating less and moving more.

Some side effects are good

Here is a cool tidbit; a nice side effect of weight training with a well-designed program is improved posture. Resistance training strengthens the muscles responsible for proper standing, sitting and walking. Better posture means higher caloric expenditure at rest, and a higher calorie burn when walking, moving around and training. Muscles responsible for good posture make up a large percentage of your muscle mass, so they burn the most energy throughout the day!

Do I need to go to the gym?

For your strength training, it's up to you whether you want to join a gym or not. I have designed the programs in this book so you can do them at home, because I want you to change your routine as little as possible. Going to the gym may not be necessary. If you look at a conventional gym, 90% of the space is taken up by machines. While you might be sharing *some* hardware with the bodybuilders and gymrats (dumbbells, barbells, and should you join a gym, machines), you certainly will not be training like bodybuilders, because you aren't bodybuilders.

Machines were invented in order to put specific stress on specific muscle necessary to stand out in the sport of bodybuilding. Apart from the occasional rehabilitation needs for special populations (disabled or hurt people), machines have little to offer compared to free weights, especially if your goal is to train for health and fitness.

Back in the day, beginners were advised to use machines rather than free weights because they lacked the skills to handle free weights, but as we found out more about the human body, we also discovered that machines can weaken small auxiliary muscles that are weak in beginners already, thus sabotaging further strength gains. Machines also fail to optimally train the neuromyofascial system – an intricate system of communication between muscles, joints and your brain, a system that controls movement in the most subtle way.

Neuromyofascial

You don't need to know this word anymore. Just like math, you will not use it again, and just like you did with math, you can now forget this, too.

Free weights present a more anatomically natural way to train, they make more muscles work at one time and don't allow for asymmetric development of body parts. It's very hard to over train and injure a muscle with free weights, as opposed to machines, and best of all, they can be portable and taken anywhere you go: home, hotel, garage, office, beach...

Can you exercise really hard and then just eat what you want?

Some people have tried to out exercise bad diets and failed miserably. To quote the title of a famous book: "You can't outrun a doughnut!" Sure, if you adhere to your diet most of the time, but fall off the wagon here and there, an exercise session will help you cushion the blow. Still, remember not to count on exercise to make up for your everyday poor nutrition. The more you exercise the more your appetite increases since your body craves quality calories for recovery. Try to feed it with junk foods and your body will be left craving even more macro and micro nutrients, thus sending more and more hungry signals that will inevitably throw you off of your desired fat burning trend, not to mention compromise your health.

Using exercise for fat loss and the hierarchy of training

Most of you will be surprised to find out that an hour of heavy training barely burns 500-600 calories, with an extra 100-200 calories spent for recovery in the following 24-48 hours. That's not a ton, so it seems almost as easy to just give up one of the two double burgers you were going to eat and call it even. Don't, because exercise is more than just calories.

The most powerful effect of strength training is that it forces the nutrients to go to the muscle when you do eat and also tells your body to spare your muscle at times when you don't have enough energy and need to pull from your reserves. This works perfectly when you are trying to lose fat because more of the food that you eat gets shunted to the muscle and much of the extra energy you need when you eat less comes from your fat stores (and not muscle). So, as a result, you lose very little, if any, lean body mass. You might even gain some muscle, all due to tweaking your style of training.

Eat and train, and keep your metabolism high

This effect is much less pronounced with aerobic training, which relies on a smaller percentage of muscle and requires less energy for any given amount of time. This is the main reason why I want you to have the strength training basics covered before you do any extra aerobic work.

When you look at your fat loss training, it will be a combination of the most important factors, followed by the ones that are not so critical. I want you to be smart, leveraging your time so that you get the most out of what time you have. Do not waste your valuable time on ineffective exercise protocols!

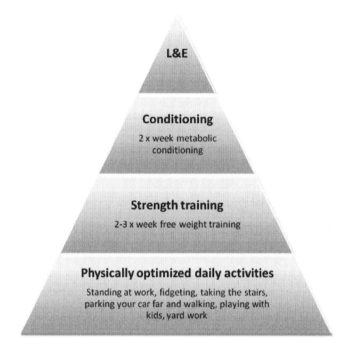

Look at this chart. At the bottom of the fat loss hierarchy, I have placed activities you do daily. Those are the activities that comprise a *huge* amount of your energy expenditure. You have seen them in your Life Questionnaire in the Life chapter. Go back and see which ones you score less than a 5, and see how you could optimize them. Could you do your own yard work? Play with the kids instead of watching TV?

Make the changes that you can. At the very least, try to do some of your work (talking on the phone, checking email, etc.) standing. Standing burns about one and a half times the calories of sitting, and ensures better posture. Sitting in chairs is actually unnatural to us, and negatively affects our muscles, blood pressure and yep, even our prostates.

Next up (higher on the list), is strength and weight training. It's higher in our hierarchy because of its power to direct the calories you consume toward muscle building and to allow your body to use body fat for energy during recovering and at rest.

If you have covered the base of the pyramid and are already living an optimized lifestyle and doing three strength workouts a week, you can consider some added conditioning work; things like sprints, intervals, and short but fast runs. The conditioning section of our book covers the basics, so your toolbox will be full of ideas and routines.

Putting your tv time to good use

Television is known by many derogatory names, but the one that I want to focus on here, is "time waster." Hey, I watch tv, too, but I've tried to find ways to put my tv time to good use.

***Foam rolling** – A foam roller is a long cylinder of hard foam that you lay on to give yourself a massage, even in front of the tv! Benefits are similar to those of a true massage, but in the privacy of your own home at a fraction of the cost. Foam rollers are becoming more and more popular in commercial gyms, and are now even available at Amazon, Target, and Walmart.*

***Stretching** – most of us could do with a little stretching of tight muscles, but who wants to put in the time? Whoever is responsible for carpet in front of 99% of the televisions was a genius!*

***Folding laundry** – this makes the wife happy*

***Food prep** – if your tv is visible from the kitchen, use this to your advantage, and get your lunches prepped while you tune in to your favorite show*

***Exercise** – depending on the room you have and the location of your television, you might find tv time to be the perfect time to do your workouts. Make sure you can concentrate enough to have good form and keep things going at the desired pace, please.*

Finally, there's leisure and entertainment (L&E), which is where most little extras fall (bowling, miniature golf, dancing, chainsaw juggling, laser tag, sex…). This is sort of a catch-all for all the other things you do that aren't just sitting around. Of course they help, but you can't typically rely on them for any significant body composition changes.

Are you ready to get moving from the Kickstart to a more advanced workout? After reading about another one of our success cases, continue on to see your next steps.

Success in the spotlight #3

Leading by example

Pastor Ryan Oddo is a good friend, and is actually our Pastor at The Bridge Church in Rancho Santa Margarita, California. It's hard to recall whether Ryan became my friend or my Pastor first, but since the two events happened within seconds of each other, why quibble?

I feel honored to have Ryan in our book, and I need to point out that, like our other success cases, we've learned a lot from him, too. From Ryan I learned to minister rather than preach, even when it comes to food and nutrition. It's amazing how much more people listen, learn, and respect when the message comes to them in a positive way. I learned *that* and...

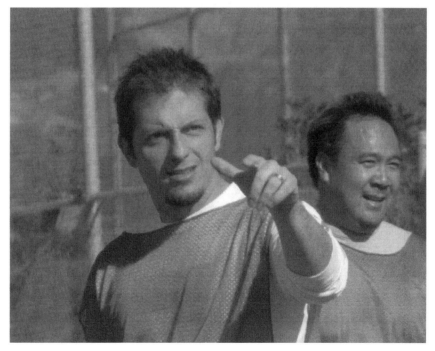

...flag football is serious business!

Pastor Ryan Oddo, 35 years old, 160 lbs, 5'7"

Ryan decided to lose some weight when he was 30 years old, and has kept it off since, inspiring others in the community to get and stay fit.

Galya – Now that you've lost the weight you wanted to lose, are you more aware of the specific issues that you had? Do you have any favorite methods to keep things in check now?

Ryan – I get heavier when I eat more good foods. My draws are bigger portions. But, I understand calories now and know how to control portions. I do one day fasts to get on track. I do liquids and fast for 24 hrs. I try to be better at the meals, but fasting clears my head and resets my attitude, it helps me regain control.

Galya – Do you have compliance problems when you fast all day? Do you tend to eat more at the next meals?

Ryan – No. I kind of *want* to eat more, but my stomach has shrunk so much I cannot eat more. I get fuller sooner.

Galya – What's different now? What did you change?

Ryan – My perception of what was happening to my body and understanding what happens to my body changed things. It was empowering to know more about calories. The satisfaction levels of carbs vs. protein. Now I know how to look at pasta vs. vegetable or cereal vs. eggs. I have been eating more protein, and when I order sides I now get veggies.

Galya – Were you active during your weight loss efforts?

Ryan – I was running two miles and doing bodyweight exercises, but I wasn't fit enough to run so much, and had gotten weak. Roland and I went to just bodyweight exercises. It got better over time until I was able to run again.

Galya – What did you do to your diet?

Ryan – I didn't exclude ANY food. I just managed it better. I had the skill to manage it now.

Galya – Did you have any friends that supported you? Did your family support you?

Ryan – My wife was very supportive. I told my wife I was taking nutrition classes and she really supported me. This also got her to stop nagging me.

Galya – What do you think made you gain weight initially?

Ryan – Not realizing how much I ate and how high calorie foods added up.

Galya – What did you change to lose weight?

Ryan – How much food to eat. Portion control.

Galya – How do you reduce the damage of non-optimal meals? Any strategies?

Ryan – A bad meal is typically either lunch or dinner. I control the type of food because I am not good at all at portion control. Also, I only snack if I have a snack on hand (jerky or nuts). I'm successful because I don't overthink things. I consider things, but I don't say "you can't have this, you can't have that." I use a check book system, where things have to balance. As long as I am not seeing the scale go up...

Galya – What stops people from losing weight?

Ryan – Not understanding calories and activity levels. They also don't start to lose weight because they don't get educated. People don't trust themselves to do it right and never start.

Galya – How did you learn?

Ryan – When I want to learn I do it through people. Go to the experts.

Galya – Thanks, Ryan. Any closing thoughts?

Ryan – It's easier when you are aware of what it takes, rather than struggling and living just on the edge. I thrive on the freedom of reality.

Ryan is the Pastor of The Bridge, in Rancho Santa Margarita, California (*thebridgersm.com*) and was kind enough to marry Galya and me in March of 2011. Ryan is a passionate figure in the church and community, a great friend, the proud father of two awesome boys, and the wonderful husband to our friend Johanna.

9

Your training plan

As I promised you in the Kickstart program, you will make training a permanent part of your lifestyle. At this point, you have either been training for a while, so you just got this book for the diet and life tips, or you are just starting out. After the Kickstart, you are now physically prepared to jump into your fat loss routine.

Training is a supplement?

Yes, whether you call it training, weightlifting, or just exercise, it is actually a supplement or substitute for the physical activity that we used to naturally do. Hunting, farming, building, walking, and running were part of our ancestors' lives, whether they wanted it to be or not. Our ancestors didn't have to lift weights to workout, run 5Ks, and swing kettlebells; their work was hard and heavy! Modern technology and lifestyles allow us to sit more and work less, which is both a benefit and a drawback, as we've now seen.

We've set up a 12 week program that will allow you to make continuous improvements in your fat loss. It's all home based, so you can do it almost anywhere; your backyard, your living room, your garage or your basement. You can exercise when you have time, and do so in the comfort of your own home.

What's special about these exercises?

Your body is designed to do a few basic movements, such as pushing, pulling, bending, twisting, and lifting. I chose exercises based on these movements; they use a large percentage of your muscle, improve your ability to move in daily life, elevate your metabolism, and expend the maximum amount of calories when worked. Sitting, driving, typing, and reading have a negative effect on our health and muscular system. The exercises in our program are specifically chosen to reverse it. They are also the safest exercise to build strength in beginners, and allow us to include harder versions of the exercises as you progress.

In addition, I don't want you to have to join a gym if you don't want to, spending extra time away from your family and extra money for a membership that you don't always need. I also don't need you to change your image to that of a gym rat, or put on fancy running gear and become one of those jogging guys. If you choose to join a gym, that's fine, but know that to be successful, you don't need to.

Since our plan is all about doing something *now*, I had you start with the Kickstart program way back near the beginning of the book, all without any preparation or new equipment. Now that we are taking things up a notch or two, you will add things to your home workout arsenal as you go. It's just one small element or tool at a time, all in accordance with the increasing difficulty of the program and your needs. These tools are not expensive, and they aren't things that you'll only use once and then store in the garage or use as a coat rack.

What kind of equipment do I need?

Your program has 3 phases, each building on the previous one, and each phase increasing in complexity and effectiveness. Each of those phases is 4-6 weeks long; four weeks if you choose to workout the optimal three times per week and six weeks if you choose to train the minimum amount of two times per week.

Each phase begins with a test of strength so that you can monitor and celebrate your progress.

Each phase will also require the purchase of an inexpensive and easy to find item for your home gym. Most of the equipment is easy to find locally or online. Check out the "Store" tab on TheFitInk.com for good online options.

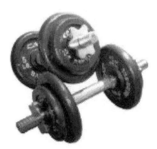

Phase 1: A set of adjustable dumbbells that go up to 40 lbs. Since this is the first phase of training after the Kickstart, I suggest you buy them now. Your local Walmart may have them. Cap Barbell has a decent set on Amazon.com. Check out the "Store" tab on TheFitInk.com for online options.

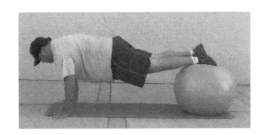

Phase 2: A Swiss ball and extra 2-4 plates for your dumbbells. Again, Walmart probably has the plates and the ball, but Amazon and Perform Better have them too. When you're looking for your Swiss ball, look for one that says it's burst resistant or burst proof. Luckily, most modern Swiss balls are made to deflate slowly, rather than pop, should something go wrong.

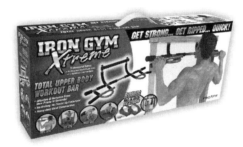

Phase 3: Pull up bar. Target, Walmart, and virtually every sporting goods store has these. I recommend the Iron Gym!

You will only buy equipment as your training needs increase, so there is no rush to make a whole or traditional home gym right now.

I don't have 30-40 minutes to get my sweat on! What do I do?

That's a great question. Your workout doesn't need to happen all at once. You can do half of your workout in the morning and half upon returning from work; just don't forget to warm up again.

Your starting point

Before you start, make sure you take your starting stats: weight, measurements, body fat percentage, and pictures; then proceed with taking the fitness test. This test shows your current level of fitness and when you take it again, you would be surprised at how much progress you have made in just 4 weeks. You can find charts to record your starting stats in the appendix.

But wait; before you do the fitness test, here is a short warm up I want you to do. If you are unfamiliar with the benefits of warmups, I briefly explain them below. If you know your stuff, proceed to the actual warmup and the fitness test

So what's a warmup?

A warmup is always a good idea, skipping it isn't. You'll see all sorts of opinions on warming up, some as extreme as not warming up at all, or stretching for half an hour before a workout. I like a warmup that is similar to the activity that will follow it.

Warming up serves a few important functions:

• It prepares your nervous system for the workout to follow, making sure you will execute movements properly and effectively.

• It primes your joints, which are not evenly lubricated due to our daily postures at work.

• It gets your brain in learning mode, allowing you to do new exercises better.

• It improves energy transport to and from the muscles.

The warm up we have designed specifically prepares small muscle groups that are weakened in everyday life to fully and healthfully participate in supporting large muscle groups for best workout effectiveness.

A warm up needn't *necessarily* involve stretching, running or the other activities that are generally considered warm ups. A proper warm up is 5-15 minutes of activities that best approximate what you will be doing *during* your workout. This is the type of warmup Galya's happy, pain free, and result driven clients do, and they love it! One big bonus; no treadmill required!

The warmup – the warmup is the same warmup that you used in the Kickstart, so you should be pretty comfortable with it, already. You can use the following table as a reminder of what to do, and flip back to Chapter Two if you need to see the warmup in action again.

Also, I encourage you to go to TheFitInk.com/ManOnTop andd download our blank workout log to record your routine and track your progress. At the very least, get out a notebook or scratch paper and write these all down, along with how many of each exercise you need to do.

Ready? Here we go!

Warmup	
Exercise	**Repetitions**
Joint Rotations	10 per joint – each side
Face the Wall Ys	10
Ankle Mobility	10 per side
Split Stance Rotations	10 per side
Pushups Plus	10
Rockbacks	10
Glute Bridges	10
Jumping Jacks	1 minute

Warmup? Done!

Well done! If this is your first time doing the warm up, the next thing you do is your Fitness Test.

The fitness test

This is not a pass/fail test. This test is a way to judge your progress as you get fitter over time. On your first day, after your warmup, you will test yourself, physically, recording your scores. After a few weeks, we're going to have you retest to see how far you've come. You might already be a stud in certain area, but you're likely going to see some solid improvement when you test yourself again!

Here are the exercises that you'll be doing in during the Fitness Test – pushups, bodyweight squats, jumping jacks, front plank, side planks, sit and reach, run, walk, or cycle.

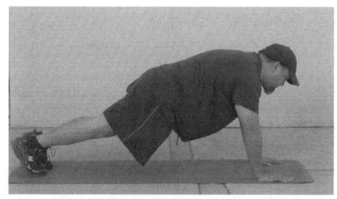

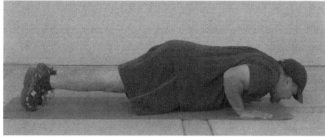

Pushups: Get in the classic pushup position, with your hands under your shoulders. Keep your abs very tight as you slowly lower yourself down, with your ankles, knees, hips, upper back and head in one straight line. Lower yourself until your shoulders are lower than your elbows and push yourself back up. Do as many as possible.

Do this basic pushup, if possible, but if you are unable to do any, you should do the Elevated Pushup, below.

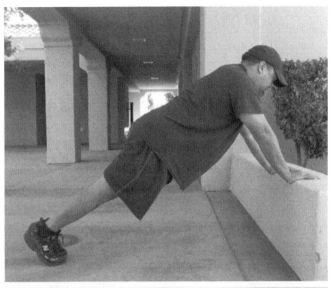

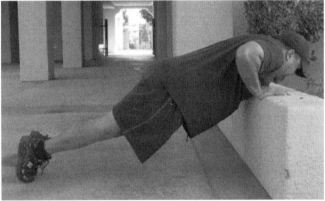

Elevated Pushups – Put your hands on the bench, chair, or wall, slightly wider than your shoulders. Straighten your body over the ground, rising up onto your toes. You will be at an angle, not flat over the floor. Keep your abs braced the entire time. The tighter your body, the more pushups you'll be able to do. Lower yourself until your chest is an inch or two from the bench or chair. Keep your body stiff and straight. Push yourself back up, pause, and repeat for as many reps as possible.

Because this pushup is done with hands on a wall or chair, it is a good choice for those who can't yet do regular pushups. Elevated Pushups may also be used later as a way to do more pushups than you could normally do. Using a bench, low wall, or sturdy chair under your hands (instead of the floor) reduces the weight that you press with your arms and chest.

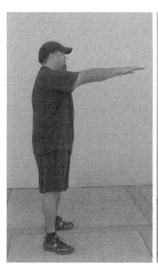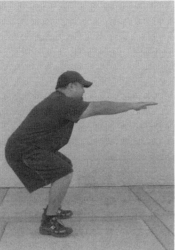

Bodyweight Squats – Stand with your feet about shoulder width, and your toes in line with your knees. Begin to squat as if you were going to sit down into a chair. Squat down as far as possible, extending your arms to counterbalance. Don't let your lower back round. Only squat as far down as you can without rounding. Push back up to a standing position, pause, and repeat.

Jumping Jacks – Start with your feet together, hands at your sides, then jump spreading your feet to just beyond shoulder width and simultaneously bring your arms up and together, then jump again, bringing your feet together again, and your arms down and to your sides. Perform Jumping Jacks for 1 minute.

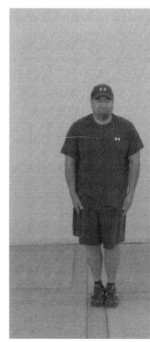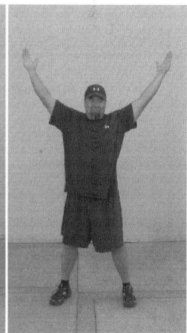

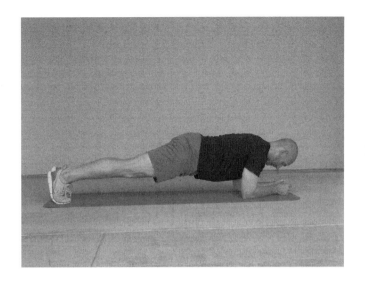

Front Planks – Get in a pushup position, and drop to your elbows, making sure your body is in one straight line from ankles through hips to neck. Do not round your upper back; rather focus on maintaining this position using your abs. Keep your butt cheeks tight and a straight lower back. Hold for as long as possible.

If you are not ready for a full Front Plank yet, you can do them on your knees, as shown below.

Front Planks, on knees – Get in a pushup position, and drop to your elbows and knees, making sure your body is in one straight line from hips to neck. Do not round your upper back; rather focus on maintaining this position using your abs. Keep your butt cheeks tight and a straight lower back. Hold for as long as possible.

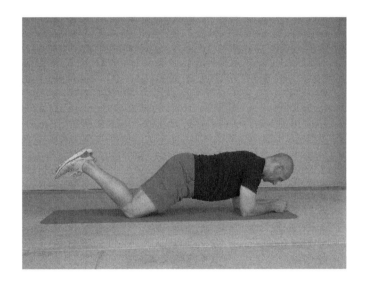

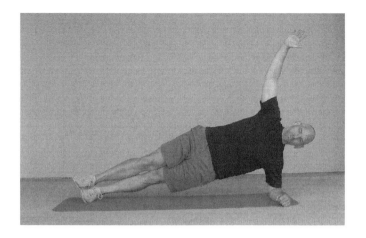

Side Planks – Lie on your side and place your elbow directly under your shoulder. Put your hips, knees, and ankles in line and push yourself up. Hold this position for as long as possible (ALAP) and then repeat on the other side.

If you are not ready for a full Side Plank yet, you can do them on your knees, as shown below.

Side Planks, on knees – Lie on your side, knees bent at a right angle, and place your elbow directly under your shoulder. Put your hips and knees in line and push yourself up. Hold this position for as long as possible (ALAP) and then repeat on the other side.

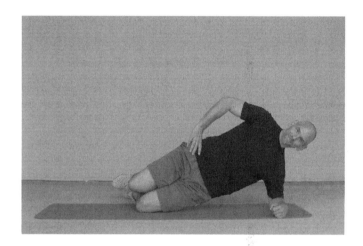

Run, walk, or cycle – not pictured, but you probably know how to do these things. Pick the exercise that you want to do or simply can do, recording the time to complete your mile. If you can't accurately measure a mile because you don't have access to a track, pedometer, GPS, etc., just do your best and make sure to use the same route the next time you test. If you are riding a stationary bike, these can easily measure your distance in miles, but it will be helpful to also record the settings you used, such as resistance, hills, etc.

Ready, set, test!

Set up a flat area free of any furniture or objects on the ground, enough to where you can freely extend your arms and legs in all directions, get up and down from the ground, assume the pushup position, etc. Get a sheet of paper and a pen or pencil ready and write down the exercises, using the following chart as reference, or download and print the forms from the website.

Also, you'll need to grab a watch or stopwatch or use one on your mobile phone, since all the exercises will require some sort of timing device. Before or after these exercises you will need to time your mile walk/run or bike time, so either look for a track to walk/run or plan to use the bike or treadmill in the local gym or fitness center.

While it's best to do the 1 mile run immediately after the rest of the workout, sometimes it's not possible, so just do your best.

Initial Fitness Test

Exercise	Required Effort	Score
Pushups	Maximum Number (in one minute)	
Bodyweight Squats	Maximum Number (in one minute)	
Jumping Jacks	Maximum Number (in one minute)	
Front Planks	Hold For Time (seconds)	
Side Planks (Right)	Hold For Time (seconds)	
Side Planks (Left)	Hold For Time (seconds)	
1 Mile Run/Walk or 3 Mile Bike or Stationary Bike	Time To Completion (minutes)	

Test complete!

Depending on your starting fitness level, the Fitness Test will leave you feeling like you had a true workout and need a deserved rest OR feeling like you can do more. If you have more in you, you can jump right into your first workout right now. If you're beat, plan your next workout for tomorrow and hit the shower.

Workout basics

In the workouts and the workout log sheets you will see sets, reps, rest, etc. Here are some brief descriptions of some of these training terms.

Reps – Reps or repetitions are the number of times you perform an exercise. Reps will also help determine the weight you use. Always use a weight that is challenging, so that you could do no more than one or two reps beyond the prescribed number of repetitions. This practice, stopping even when you know you could get one or two more reps in, is called "leaving some in the tank," and helps to keep injury and overtraining at bay. Don't worry, grinding them out and muscle failure has been shown to *decrease* strength, not increase it!

Make sure you use more weight when you see fewer repetitions prescribed and less weight when the reps are high in number. When an exercise changes from 12 reps to 10, you also need to increase the weight used. Also, consider increasing the weight when things get easy and you feel like you are leaving three reps in the tank, rather than just one or two.

Sets – Sets are groups of repetitions separated with a rest break.

Circuit – A circuit is a sequence of exercises done in a row. A circuit can be done once, or may be repeated after a short rest period.

AMRAP – As Many Reps As Possible. Start your set and keep going until you can't do another rep with good form. If you feel like you could just squeeze out another one or two reps, that's the time to stop. Don't go until complete failure.

ALAP – As Long As Possible. Hold the exercise position until you can no longer maintain it, and your form starts to slip or sag. Don't go until complete failure.

Rest – You will rest a different amount of time depending on the phase of your program. Try to get close to the prescribed rest period, but don't stress about hitting it perfectly.

Glutes – This is short for gluteus, and is merely exercise lingo for the muscles of your butt.

How heavy should I go?

Another great question. In order to get the most from your training, it's important to challenge your muscles, but not destroy them.

• Choose a weight that allows you to do all reps with good form. If you feel like you could have kept going and going, then you need to increase the weight. On the other hand, if you are supposed to do ten and you fail to lift it eight times OR the last rep or two is really ugly and a struggle, you went too heavy.

• When you are doing a strength workout, it's generally good to leave one or two reps "in the tank." This means that you don't push yourself to muscular failure, but stop when your form starts to go out the window. This tends to happen when you could still push out one or two more, but your form would suffer.

• If you realize that you are lifting too light or too heavy, change on the next set if you can. You don't have to wait until the next time you train.

• If you feel really strong or really weak, adjust the weight up or down for this training session. Getting stronger is a long term proposition, and your strength naturally ebbs and flows. This is another good reason why it's good to leave a few "in the tank," so you don't have to be perfect and just barely grind out that last rep.

Fat Loss Workouts

Phase 1

Number of workouts: 12 (six A and six B workouts)

Workout frequency: 2-3 times per week. Always allow at least one day in between workouts.

Equipment: an exercise mat or towel and an adjustable dumbbell set of about 40lbs. See Appendix 4 for sources of your equipment.

Time for completion: ~35 minutes

For this phase, you will alternate between workouts A and B. Do one, take at least one day's break and then do the other one for a total of 12 workouts.

All exercises will be done in a circuit.

Workout A

Always allow at least one day of rest between Workout A and Workout B.

Let's start with the warmup

Warmup	
Exercise	**Repetitions**
Joint Rotations	10 per joint – each side
Face the Wall Ys	10
Ankle Mobility	10 per side
Split Stance Rotations	10 per side
Pushups Plus	10
Rockbacks	10
Glute Bridges	10
Jumping Jacks	1 minute

And now to the real workout!

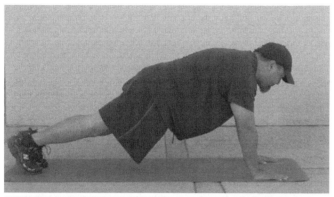

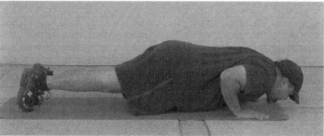

Pushups – Put your hands on the floor, slightly wider than your shoulders. Straighten your body over the ground, rising up onto your toes. Keep your abs braced the entire time. The tighter your body, the more pushups you'll be able to do. Lower until your chest is an inch or two from the floor. Keep your body stiff and straight. Push yourself back up, pause, repeat.

Here we show two versions of the pushup: the classic pushup, and with feet elevated on the next page. Once you can do more than 15 classic pushups, it's time to elevate your feet, using the Feet Elevated Pushups.

Feet Elevated Pushups: Use a step or your stairs to elevate your feet. Put your hands on the floor, slightly wider than your shoulders. Keep your abs braced the entire time. The tighter your body, the more pushups you'll be able to do. Lower until your chest is an inch or two from the floor. Keep your body stiff and straight. Push yourself back up, pause, repeat.

The higher you set your feet, the harder it gets. If you can't do eight "classic" pushups yet, use the Elevated Pushup shown early in the "Fitness Test."

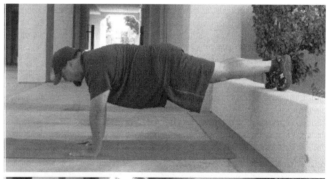

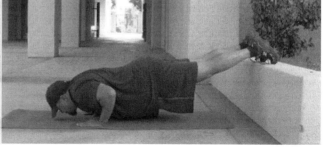

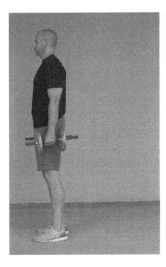
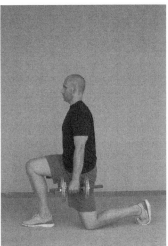

Reverse Lunges with Dumbbells: Hold a pair of dumbbells at your sides. Stand with your feet at hip width. Step back with one foot. Lower your body until your knees reach 90 degrees. Keep your back straight and your abs braced. Pause and push yourself back to the starting position

Bentover Y and T Raises: Get in a wide bent over stance, keeping your back straight. Drop your arms straight at the floor and raise them up in a Y shape, thumbs up style, using the muscles between your shoulder blades, then drop them down and raise them straight to the side, thumbs pointing at the floor. Do 5 of each and add small weight plates if you need to.

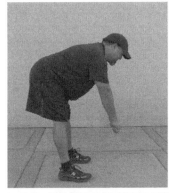
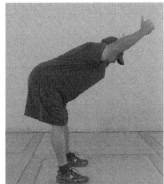
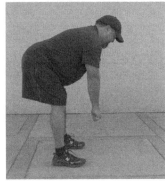
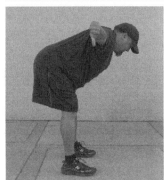

Dumbbell Romanian Deadlifts: Hold two dumbbells in front of your thighs with your palms facing you. Pull your shoulder blades together and keep your upper back tight. Bend at the hips and push them back, lowering your torso until it's almost parallel with the ground. To return to the starting position, squeeze your glutes and push your hips forward.

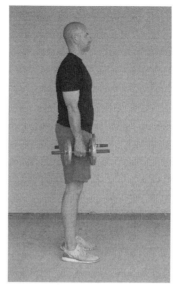 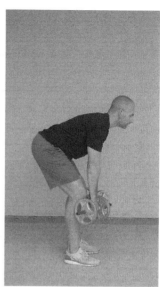

Back saver tip

To make sure you are bending at the hips during these exercises, and not bending your lower back, check your form with the following trick: get on your knees with a broomstick behind your back. Get it in contact with the back of your head, upper back and pelvis. Hinge from your hips, pushing your butt backward. Squeeze your glutes to get yourself back up. Make sure the stick is in contact with all three points at all times.

This same movement transfers to standing exercises, so try it on your feet, too.

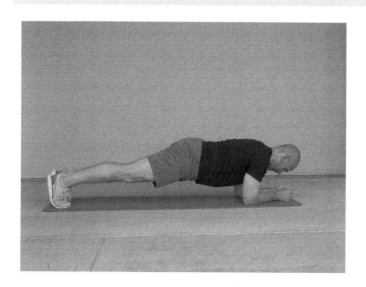

Front Planks – Get in a pushup position, and drop to your elbows, making sure your body is in one straight line from ankles through hips to neck. Do not round your upper back; rather focus on maintaining this position using your abs. Keep your butt cheeks tight and a straight lower back. Hold for as long as possible.

If you are not ready for a full Front Plank yet, you can do them on your knees, as shown in the Kickstart.

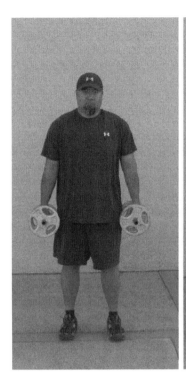 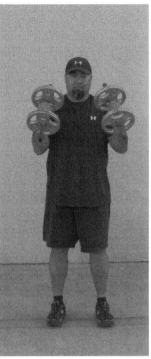

Hammer Curls: Stand straight or with your back to a wall, holding the dumbbells in a neutral grip (think of how you would hold a hammer). Curl them up, making sure your elbows stay as stable as possible. Lower twice as slow as you lift the weights.

How do I log my workouts?

You can use a simple notebook or composition book, an Excel spreadsheet, or even print out the workout templates from TheFitInk.com/ManOnTop to chart the weight or reps progress.

Phase 1

Workout A — 6 Workouts

Do in a circuit, resting 1 minute after each circuit **Exercise**	*Workouts 1-6* **Sets X Reps**
Pushups (or Elevated Pushups)	3 X AMRAP
Dumbbell Reverse Lunges	3 X 8-10
Prone Y And Ts	3 X 5 Each
Dumbbell Romanian Deadlifts	3 X 8-10
Front Planks	3 X ALAP
Hammer Curls	3 X 8-10
* AMRAP = As Many As Possible, ALAP = As Long As Possible	

Workout B

Always allow at least one day of rest between Workout A and Workout B.

Again, we always start with the warmup

Warmup	
Exercise	**Repetitions**
Joint Rotations	10 per joint – each side
Face the Wall Ys	10
Ankle Mobility	10 per side
Split Stance Rotations	10 per side
Pushups Plus	10
Rockbacks	10
Glute Bridges	10
Jumping Jacks	1 minute

Warmup? Done, and now, on to the exercises!

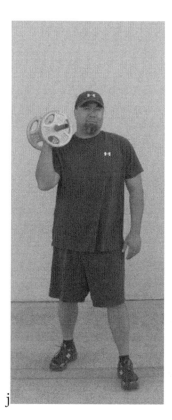
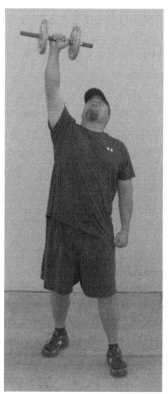

Shoulder Side Presses: Take a wide boxing stance, one foot slightly in front of the other, and hold a dumbbell at the shoulder. Contract your shoulder blade to give your shoulder a stable support to push from and press the weight up, pause, and lower it under control. Keep your abs braced the whole time. Do eight reps, then switch arms and legs and repeat on the other side.

Goblet Squats: Stand with your feet at shoulder width and hold a dumbbell in both hands at chest level. Sit far back until your thighs reach parallel, keeping your back straight. Use your glutes to push yourself up.

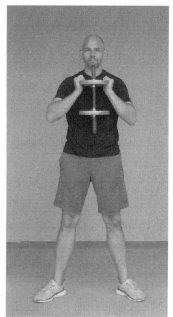
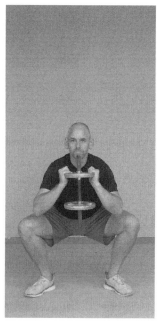

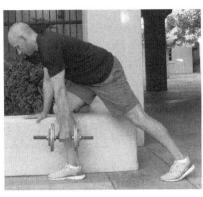 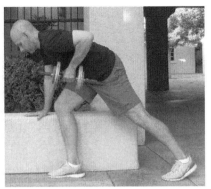

Dumbbell Rows:
Assume a bent over position, with one foot slightly in front of the other, and the hand on the same side resting on a bench, wall, or chair. Extend your free arm to grab a dumbbell. Keeping your back neutral, row the weight up using the muscles between your shoulder blades. Hold for a second and lower slowly, repeating for all reps. Switch sides, and repeat for the opposite arm.

One Leg Glute bridges – Lie on your back and bend your knees. Bring one knee to your chest. Lift your butt off the floor, squeezing your glute as hard as you can and making sure you are not using the back of your leg or your lower back to lift yourself up.

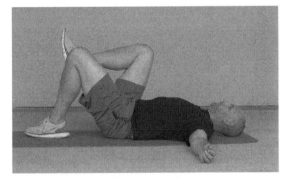

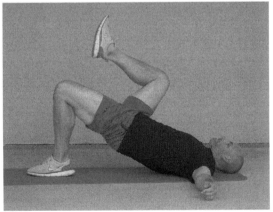

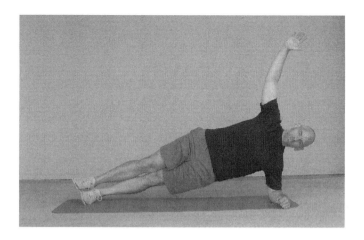

Side Planks – Lie on your side and place your elbow directly under your shoulder. Put your hips, knees, and ankles in line and push yourself up. Hold this position for as long as possible (ALAP) and then repeat on the other side.

If you are not ready for a full Side Plank yet, you can do them on your knees, as shown in the Kickstart.

Standing French Presses: Stand and hold a dumbbell in both hands above your head. Bend your arms at the elbows until you get the dumbbell low behind your head. Contract your triceps and push the weight back up until your arms are straight overhead and fully extended.

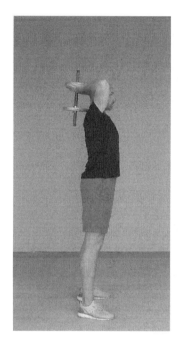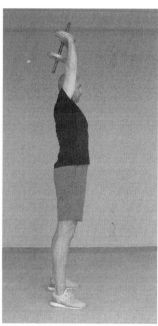

Phase 1

Workout B — 6 Workouts

Do in a circuit, resting 1 minute after each circuit	Workouts 1-6
Exercise	**Sets X Reps**
Shoulder Side Presses	3x 8
Goblet Squats	3 X 8
Dumbbell Rows	3 X 8-10
One Leg Glute Bridges	3x 10
Side Planks	3 X ALAP
Standing French Presses	3 X 8-10
* AMRAP = As Many As Possible, ALAP = As Long As Possible	

Good job. You have made it to Phase 2. That means you should now buy your Swiss ball and at least 20 extra pounds to add to your adjustable dumbbell sets. If you have found out that you are a lot stronger than that please do not hesitate to grab as much weight as you need, since you will be getting even stronger in this next phase.

Fitness Test

It's now time to repeat the fitness test you did at the beginning of phase 1 and record the changes in your performance.

Fitness Test After Phase 1		
Exercise	**Required Effort**	**Score**
Pushups	Maximum Number (in one minute)	
Bodyweight Squats	Maximum Number (in one minute)	
Jumping Jacks	Maximum Number (in one minute)	
Front Planks	Hold For Time (seconds)	
Side Planks (Right)	Hold For Time (seconds)	
Side Planks (Left)	Hold For Time (seconds)	
1 Mile Run/Walk or 3 Mile Bike or Stationary Bike	Time To Completion (minutes)	

I would love to hear about your progress, so please get in touch so I can share your successes with others following the program! My email address is rdenzel@gmail.com, or you can find Galya and me on Facebook at Facebook.com/TheFitInk. I hope you'll stop by and say hi.

Phase 2

Number of workouts: 12 (six strength A and six metabolic B workouts)

Workout frequency: 2-3 times per week. Always allow at least one day in between workouts.

Equipment needed: adjustable dumbbell set with the extra weight if you need it, a Swiss ball, and an exercise mat. See Appendix 4 for sources of your equipment.

Time for completion: ~40-45 minutes

You will be alternating between workouts A and B, taking at least a day in between, for at least 12 workouts.

Workout A

Always allow at least one day of rest between Workout A and Workout B.

Let's start with the warmup

By now, the warmup should be familiar to you. You're probably getting pretty good at it, but here are the exercises, again.

Warmup	
Exercise	**Repetitions**
Joint Rotations	10 per joint – each side
Face the Wall Ys	10
Ankle Mobility	10 per side
Split Stance Rotations	10 per side
Pushups Plus	10
Rockbacks	10
Glute Bridges	10
Jumping Jacks	1 minute

Again, the warmup is complete and it's on to the main exercises!

Single Dumbbell Split Squat:
Hold one dumbbell in one hand. Step
forward with the opposite leg. Think
of your feet being aligned as if you are
stepping on two parallel train tracks.
Stand tall, bend both knees and
slowly lower yourself down until your
front thigh reaches parallel. Push
yourself up with your glutes. Make
sure your knees point at your toes at
all times.

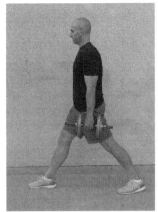 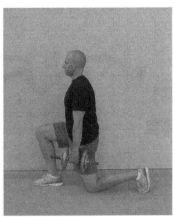

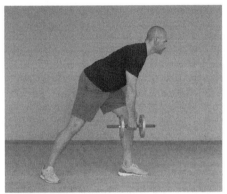

Two Point Dumbbell Rows: Assume a bent
over position, with left foot forward. Hold a
dumbbell in your right hand. Row the weight up
leading with the muscles between your shoulder
blades. Hold for a second and lower slowly,
repeating for all reps. Switch sides, and repeat for
the opposite arm.

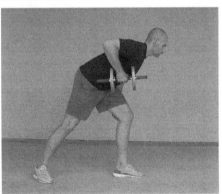

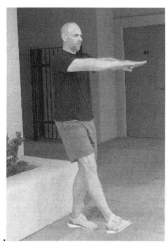 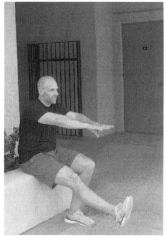

One Leg Squats to Bench: Stand in front of a bench or chair and extend one leg forward. Extend your arms, and sit back and down. Stand back up using your glutes. If you cannot do 6, do as many as you can and work your way up as you get stronger.

1 Arm Swiss Ball Presses: Lay on your Swiss ball with a dumbbell in one hand. Start by driving your elbow to the side to about 45 degrees from your body. Stabilize the ball by pushing down with your torso. Press the weight up, until your elbow is locked and then lower it down until your wrist is even with your shoulder, making sure your abs are braced and keeping you firmly on the ball. Repeat for all reps before switching sides.

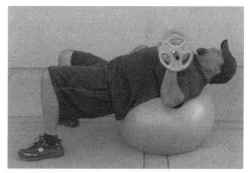

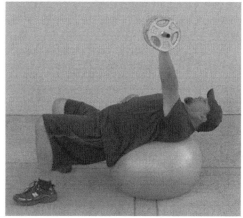

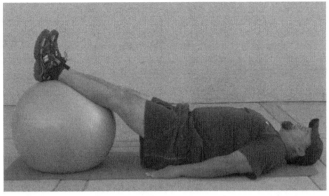

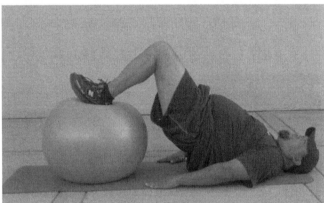

SHELCs – SHELC is short for supine hip extension with leg curl. Lie on your back and place the back of your feet and calves on a Swiss ball. Lift your hips up and while keeping your glutes tight and your body straight, roll the ball towards you. Hold for 2 seconds and slowly return to the starting position. If you find that 6 repetitions with two legs is easy, do a one leg version of the exercise, keeping your free leg up.

Mountain Climbers with 5 sec hold – Get in a pushup position. Bring one knee to your chest and contract your abs. Hold for 5 seconds and return to the pushup position. Alternate legs until you've completed all reps.

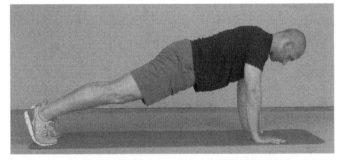

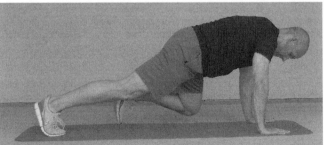

Phase 2

Workout A — Strength — 6 Workouts

Do in a circuit, resting 2 minutes after each circuit	Workouts 1-6
Exercise	**Sets X Reps**
1 Dumbbell Split Squats	*4 X 6*
2 Point Dumbbell Rows	*4 X 6*
One Leg Squats to Bench	*4 X 6*
One Arm Swiss Ball Presses	*4 X 6*
SHELCs	*4 X 8 - 12*
Mountain Climbers (with 5 second hold)	*4 X 4 – 5 Per Side*
* AMRAP = As Many As Possible, ALAP = As Long As Possible	

Workout B

Always allow at least one day of rest between Workout A and Workout B.

Again with the warmup?

Same warmup, same purpose. Let's get started!

Warmup	
Exercise	**Repetitions**
Joint Rotations	10 per joint – each side
Face the Wall Ys	10
Ankle Mobility	10 per side
Split Stance Rotations	10 per side
Pushups Plus	10
Rockbacks	10
Glute Bridges	10
Jumping Jacks	1 minute

Again, the warmup is complete and it's on to the main exercises!

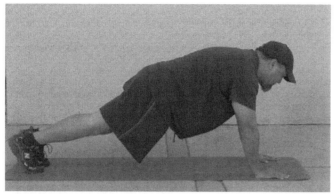

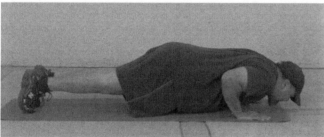

Pushups: Get in the classic pushup position, with your hands under your shoulders. Keep your abs very tight as you slowly lower yourself down, with your ankles, knees, hips, upper back and head in one straight line. Lower yourself until your shoulders are lower than your elbows and push yourself back up. Do as many as possible.

If you can do more than 15, do the Feet Elevated Pushups, below.

Feet Elevated Pushups: Use a step or your stairs to elevate your feet. Put your hands on the floor, slightly wider than your shoulders. Keep your abs braced the entire time. The tighter your body, the more pushups you'll be able to do. Lower until your chest is an inch or two from the floor. Keep your body stiff and straight. Push yourself back up, pause, repeat.

The higher you set your feet, the harder it gets. If you can't do eight "classic" pushups yet, use the Elevated Pushup shown early in the "Fitness Test."

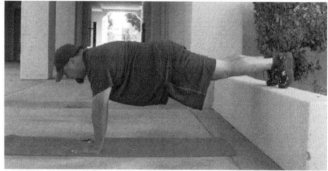

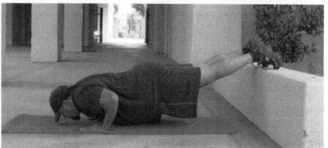

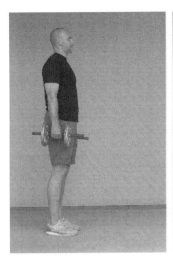 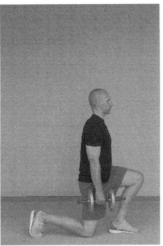

Forward Lunges with Dumbbells: Stand with your feet at hip width, holding dumbbells at your sides. Take a step forward, bending both knees until they reach 90 degrees. Use your front foot to push yourself back to the starting position. Do all reps with one leg, then switch.

Dumbbell Face Pulls: Bend over with dumbbells in your hands. Keeping your back straight, raise the weights towards the sides of your head, elbows pointing out, thinking of the same motion you do when you put sunglasses on. Use your shoulder blades to generate the movement. Pause for 1 second on top and repeat.

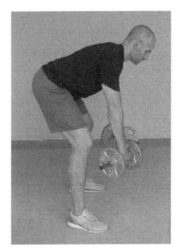 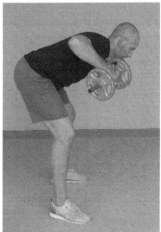

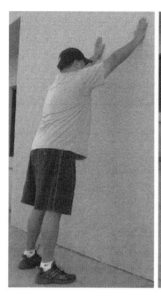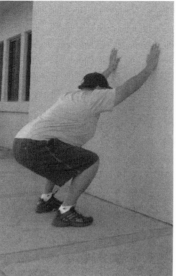

Face the Wall Squats: Stand facing a wall, toes about two feet away. Stretch your arms up, and place your palms on the wall. Start sitting back as if you are sitting into a chair, keeping your back straight and sliding your palms down the wall. Go back as far as is comfortable into a squat position. To come back up, squeeze your glutes and push off your heels, returning to the starting point. Pause, and repeat.

Hammer Curls to Press: Stand and hold two dumbbells in a hammer grip. Choose a weight that you can curl for all reps. Curl the weights up, pause at the shoulder, and press them straight overhead. Repeat.

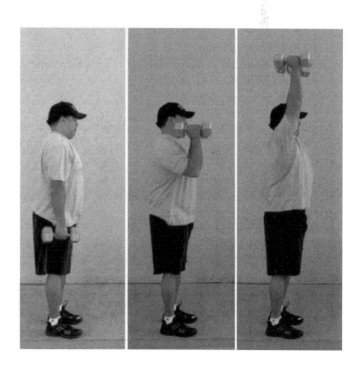

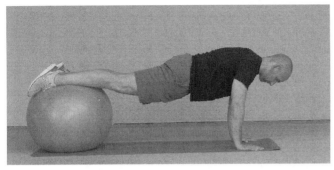

Swiss Ball Jackknives: Get in a pushup position with your lower legs on a Swiss ball. Keeping your back straight and your abs tight, pull your knees in and roll the ball toward your chest. Slowly reverse the movement and repeat.

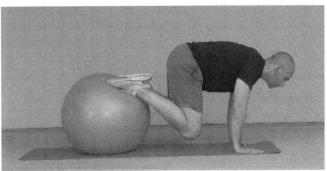

Phase 2	
Workout B — Endurance — 6 Workouts	
Do in a circuit, resting 1 minute after each circuit **Exercise**	*Workouts* *1-6* **Sets X Reps**
Pushups	3 X AMRAP
Forward Lunges w/Dumbbells	3 X 12 Per Leg
Dumbbell Face Pulls	3 X 12
Face The Wall Squats	3 X 12
Hammer Curls To Press	3 X 12
Jackknives	3 X AMRAP
* AMRAP = As Many As Possible, ALAP = As Long As Possible	

After you've done each workout six times, alternating between A and B, it's time to move on to Phase 3.

...but not before you check yourself by running through the Fitness Test again!

Fitness Test

Take at least a day off from working out, then see how you do.

Fitness Test After Phase 2		
Exercise	**Required Effort**	**Score**
Pushups	Maximum Number (in one minute)	
Bodyweight Squats	Maximum Number (in one minute)	
Jumping Jacks	Maximum Number (in one minute)	
Front Planks	Hold For Time (seconds)	
Side Planks (Right)	Hold For Time (seconds)	
Side Planks (Left)	Hold For Time (seconds)	
1 Mile Run/Walk or 3 Mile Bike or Stationary Bike	Time To Completion (minutes)	

Again, please share your progress; I'd love to hear from you on Facebook (Facebook.com/TheFitInk) or email (rdenzel@gmail.com).

Phase 3

Congratulations! You are now fitter and stronger, and as you see, it's not that hard to make exercise a part of your life!

Let's see what phase 3 has in store for you!

Number of workouts: 12 (6 strength A and 6 metabolic B workouts)

Workout frequency: 2-3 times per week. Always allow at least one day in between workouts.

Equipment: adjustable dumbbell set/Swiss ball/exercise mat/pull up bar. See Appendix 4 for sources of your equipment.

Time for completion: ~45 minutes

You will be alternating between workouts A and B, taking at least a day in between, for at least 12 workouts.

Workout A

Always allow at least one day of rest between Workout A and Workout B.

Let's start with the warmup

By now, the warmup should be familiar to you. You're probably getting pretty good at it, but here are the exercises, again.

Warmup	
Exercise	**Repetitions**
Joint Rotations	10 per joint – each side
Face the Wall Ys	10
Ankle Mobility	10 per side
Split Stance Rotations	10 per side
Pushups Plus	10
Rockbacks	10
Glute Bridges	10
Jumping Jacks	1 minute

And now to Workout A's exercises!

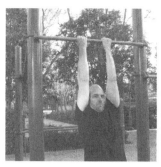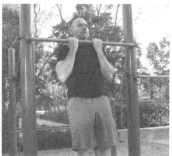

Chinups: Grab your pullup bar with an underhand grip, and hang freely, keeping your abs tight. Pull your shoulder blades down and together following through with your arms. Hold at the top position for a second, and then lower yourself down slowly. Avoid using momentum.

If 5 chinups is too much, do as many as you can, then jump and just lower yourself down for the rest of the set (also known as negative repetitions). If 5 chinups is too easy, you can always hold a dumbbell between your feet for extra weight.

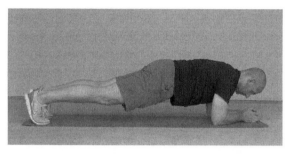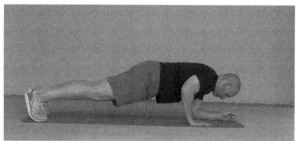

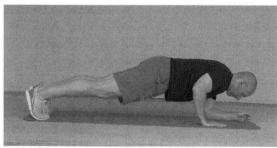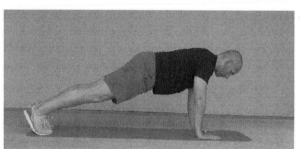

Plank to pushup: Get in a plank position on elbows and toes with your spine neutral and your head, shoulder blades, and hips in line. Keeping your abs tight, push yourself up with one hand, following with the other until you are in the top of a pushup position. Reverse the steps, dropping down to one elbow, then the other. Do all reps starting with the left, then with the right.

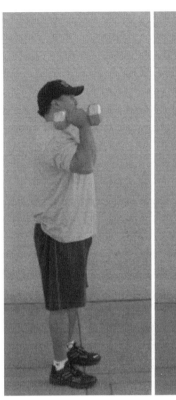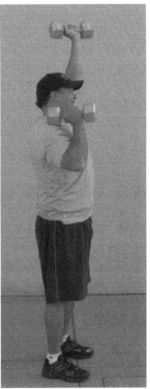

Alternating Dumbbell Presses:
Grab two dumbbells and place them in front of your shoulders. Inhale and push one up, keeping the other one ready to go. As you lower your first dumbbell down push the other one up, meeting them halfway. Repeat for all reps.

Where can I do my chinups?

You can buy a pullup bar at most sporting goods stores, Amazon.com, Walmart, and Target, then just hook it in your doorway. Most of them require no tools and use something I'll call "physics" to hang there. You could also buy one to bolt to a stud or support beam in your garage, but that would require actual work. You can also use a bar in the park near your house, a school playground, or a branch on a tree in your back yard. Just make sure it will hold you before you jump up there. You can also attach a rope to a tree in your backyard and climb it like Tarzan, but what would the neighbors say?

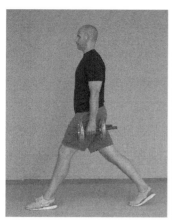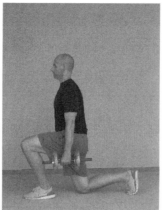

Two Dumbbell Split Squats:
Stand with one leg forward and with dumbbells at your sides. Lower yourself down, until your knees reach 90 degrees. Push up through the front heel and return to starting position. Do all reps on one side, then switch.

Dumbbell Romanian Deadlifts:
Hold two dumbbells in front of your thighs with your palms facing you. Pull your shoulder blades together and keep your upper back tight. Bend at the hips and push them back, lowering your torso until it's almost parallel with the ground. To return to the starting position, squeeze your glutes and push your hips forward.

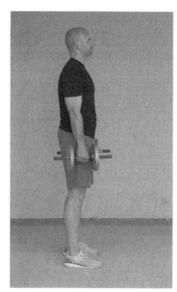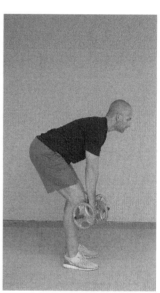

Phase 3	
Workout A — Strength — 6 Workouts	
Do in a circuit, resting 1 minute after each circuit **Exercise**	*Workouts* *1-6* **Sets X Reps**
Chinups	5 X AMAP
Alternating Dumbbell Press	5 X 5
Dumbbell Split Squat	5 X 5
Plank To Push Up	5 X AMAP Per Side
Dumbbell Romanian Deadlift	5 X 5
* AMRAP = As Many As Possible, ALAP = As Long As Possible	

Workout B

Always allow at least one day of rest between Workout A and Workout B.

Here's your warmup

Warmup	
Exercise	**Repetitions**
Joint Rotations	10 per joint – each side
Face the Wall Ys	10
Ankle Mobility	10 per side
Split Stance Rotations	10 per side
Pushups Plus	10
Rockbacks	10
Glute Bridges	10
Jumping Jacks	1 minute

And now, on to the exercises for Workout B.

Alternating Dumbbell Rows:
Bend over holding two dumbbells.
Row one dumbbell toward your
chest using the muscles of your
shoulder blades. As you return the
first dumbbell to the starting
position, row the second one up,
alternating for all reps, like a
seesaw. Keep your abs tight and
your back neutral.

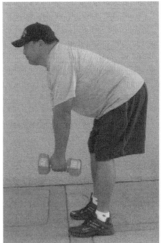
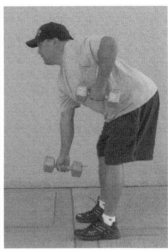

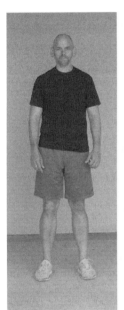
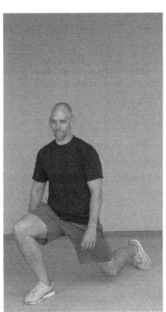
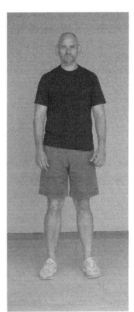
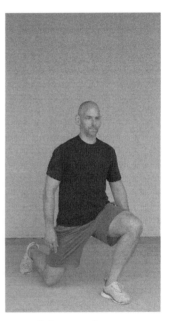

Diagonal Lunges: Stand with your feet at hip width. Take a step out and forward at a 45
degree angle. Lower yourself until both knees reach 90 degrees. Push yourself back to the
starting position. Do all reps on one side, then switch.

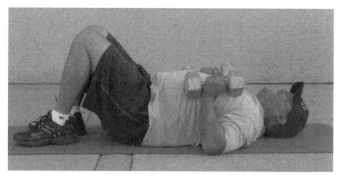

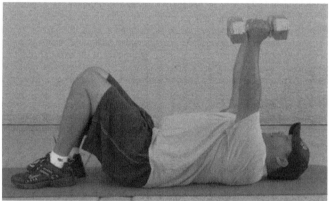

Floor presses: Get on your back and push your dumbbells up above your shoulders. Lower them down, until your elbows touch the floor and then push back up.

Dumbbell Romanian Deadlifts: Hold two dumbbells in front of your thighs with your palms facing you. Pull your shoulder blades together and keep your upper back tight. Bend at the hips and push them back, lowering your torso until it's almost parallel with the ground. To return to the starting position, squeeze your glutes and push your hips forward.

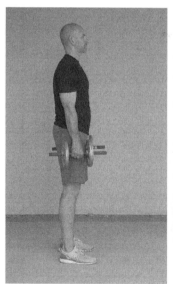
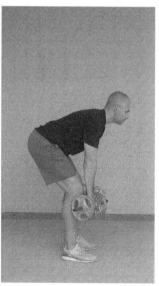

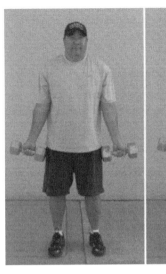 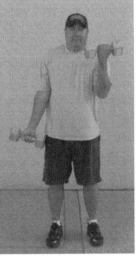

Alternating Bicep Curls: Stand and hold the dumbbells with palms facing forward.

Curl them up, one by one, alternating. Make sure your elbows stay as far back and as stable as possible.

Lower the weights twice as slow as you lift, and repeat for all reps.

Dynamic Side Planks: Lie on your side and place your elbow under your shoulder for support.

Push yourself up with your obliques until your ankles, hips, and shoulders are in a straight line above the ground.

Lower yourself down and repeat for all reps on that side before switching sides.

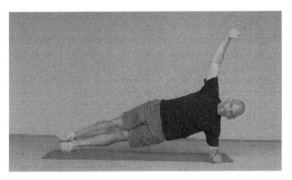

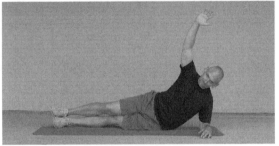

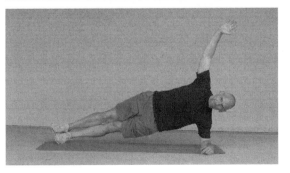

Phase 3

Workout B — Endurance — 6 Workouts

Do in a circuit, resting 1 minute after each circuit **Exercise**	Workouts 1-6 **Sets X Reps**
Chinups	5 X AMAP
Alternating Dumbbell Press	5 X 5
Dumbbell Split Squat	5 X 5
Plank To Push Up	5 X AMAP Per Side
Dumbbell Romanian Deadlift	5 X 5
* AMRAP = As Many As Possible, ALAP = As Long As Possible	

Congratulations! You've completed all phases of this program, and you just have one final Fitness Test to complete. Take a few days rest before taking the Fitness Test.

After the Test, take a hard earned rest week, take a read through our resources section, and pick your next program! Your body just gets better from here on out!

When you're feeling tired or beat up

Being successful at managing your weight requires being active, paying attention to your nutrition, and managing your life, but many people forget that all of this can be tiring. When you don't sleep enough, you don't have the energy to be as active as you like during the day, and your workouts suffer, slowing your progress.

Instead of forcing yourself to train, acknowledge that you need to rest and recuperate, instead. Use a day or two to invest in your recovery with one or more of the following:

- **Sleep more** *–turn of the television and computer, dim the lights, and go to bed an hour early.*

- **Rest more** *– take extra days between workouts, and instead of adding another day of lifting, dial that back and go for a walk, instead. Take time out to read a good book on fitness, such as the latest in our friend Lou Schuler's New Rules of Lifting series.*

- **Get a massage** *– even though it sounds like a mother's day gift for your wife, keep in mind that true athletes rely on massage to speed recovery between practices and games. It will give your body the equivalent of a mini-workout, but you're not doing the work.*

- **Hot tub** *–chilling in the hot tub with your favorite refreshment relaxes the body and the mind, preparing you for a good night's sleep.*

- **Foam roll** *– A foam roller is a long cylinder of hard foam that you lay on to give yourself a massage, even in front of the tv! Benefits are similar to those of a true massage, but in the privacy of your own home at a fraction of the cost. Foam rollers are becoming more and more popular in commercial gyms, and are now even available at Amazon, Target, and Walmart.*

The Final Fitness Test – Even more awesome!

At the end of this phase, take a few days off, and then go back to the fitness test you did at the beginning of each phase, and do it one more time. Record your new scores and congratulate yourself on progressing.

Fitness Test After Phase 3

Exercise	Required Effort	Score
Pushups	Maximum Number (in one minute)	
Bodyweight Squats	Maximum Number (in one minute)	
Jumping Jacks	Maximum Number (in one minute)	
Front Planks	Hold For Time (seconds)	
Side Planks (Right)	Hold For Time (seconds)	
Side Planks (Left)	Hold For Time (seconds)	
1 Mile Run/Walk or 3 Mile Bike or Stationary Bike	Time To Completion (minutes)	

Let us know how you did! Please. Seriously.

10

Conditioning and low level exercise

It's better to burn ~~out~~ fat than to fade away

I jogged my way from 235 pounds, straight down to about 185. When I got there, I was still pretty chubby, despite losing fifty pounds. I lost more than just fat along the way; I lost muscle tissue, right along with it, going from fat to skinny fat.

Too much of the long slow jogging, "cardio," and other moderately slow endurance activities encourage the body to be lighter, which should be a good thing. But "lighter" isn't discriminating enough when you consider that there is no physiological advantage to having a lot of muscle tissue when jogging. In fact, muscle is heavier than fat for its size and takes more energy to keep around, so your body doesn't want or need it when it comes to "cardio." For this reason, traditional cardio isn't a large part of the hierarchy of fat loss. It has its place, in moderation, but it should never take the place of strength training.

You do remember the hierarchy of fat loss training, right? At the bottom, you have your physically optimized daily activities: such as walking your dog, playing with the kids, taking the stairs instead of the elevator and all that stuff. By moving more throughout your day, you guarantee that you keep using your muscle, you are burning more calories, burning more calories *from fat,* and keeping your metabolism and your energy levels high.

On the next level up, you have strength training, which is everything that you have been doing with our fat loss workout programs or your own strength training routine in the gym. Once you can ensure that you are doing those 3 times a week, feel free to go to the next level, conditioning.

For the purposes of this program, conditioning will be all non-strength training activities and even some training that might use weights or your own bodyweight for resistance. The way these are done means that they can't replace strength training, and will be done on separate days.

You will see that "conditioning" exercises go from low intensity walking to high intensity sprints and very intense weight training circuits. I encourage you to mix things up from week to week, ensuring that your body gets better conditioned, but doesn't adapt to any one exercise, reducing its effectiveness when it comes to fat burning.

You can choose to do conditioning exercises if you have the extra time AND you feel like you should be moving more than you are from your strength training and daily activity alone. You can also include them in phases 2 and 3 of your fat loss training to speed up your fat loss. I encourage you to choose the types of conditioning that you enjoy, so let's go over some of the more common options for doing aerobic activity.

Walking

Pros: Walking is easy and you can do it anywhere. It works your whole body, but mostly your hips and torso. It can really help with postural issues, and if you get your head aligned over your upper body, focus on breathing and push off with your glutes, it can really benefit your skeletal health. To recap: head aligned, ribcage relaxed, arms swinging back, push off with glutes, feet pointed forward.

Cons: You need to walk a long time to burn a significant amount of calories. Unless you are walking properly it can cause aches and pains. Your body is very adapted to walking, so it's easy for it to burn fewer and fewer calories on the same walking program. Ultimately, to keep getting greater fat loss results with walking is challenging. Consider hiking as an upgrade.

Jogging or running

I prefer shorter runs and even shorter sprints to the longer jogs, but where does one stop and the other start? Is it semantics? Only you know if you are jogging or running, but try to run whenever possible. If you find yourself out for a jog and can't bump up to a run or sprint, consider just walking instead.

Pros: almost anyone can do it (or thinks they can). Burns moderate to high calories, works your whole body.

Cons: you need to be physically fit and well aligned to run in order to avoid injury to tendons ligaments and joints. It is potentially bad for you if you are still heavy, out of shape, and just head out to the street and run. Main victims of running are knees and lower backs, necks, and sometimes even the shoulders. The body will quickly become accustomed to it which forces you to go longer distances, potentially increasing your risk of overuse injury.

Cycling

Pros: it's easy and almost anyone can do it. It can burn a lot of calories if you keep the intensity high via speed and inclines.

Cons: it won't do your posture much good since it exacerbates poor sitting and driving mechanics that you're already experiencing. It can be hard to be outside and biking in poor weather conditions.

Stationary bike

Pros: It's a cheap piece of equipment that allows you to monitor speed, distance, calories, and even more complicated data like RPMs and METs. This lets you progress in your workouts even if you want to do it in front of your TV. Others in your household might like to use it too. It is very good for high intensity interval training, the most effective form of aerobic/anaerobic training.

Cons: it shares the cons of road biking, except that it's more boring.

Elliptical trainer

Pros: it is a good piece of equipment that allows you to exercise in the comfort of your home or gym. The motion takes you out of your desk bound position, and if you pay attention to alignment it is a great form of aerobic exercise. Because of the computerized nature, you can see the data that lets you progress toward goals of speed, distance or calories burned. It is very good for high intensity interval training, the most effective form of aerobic/anaerobic training.

Cons: it could be uncomfortable due to specific body dynamics and it can stress feet and ankles too much. At home, it can be bulky and take a lot of space. Good ellipticals tend to be costly.

Treadmill

Pros: it's the closest you can get to walking or running, but you can do it inside. Works your whole body and you can adjust speed to keep intensity up as you get tired, something you cannot do outside. You can burn a moderate to high amount of calories.

Cons: good treadmills are very costly and bad treadmills can pose unnecessary stress to your joints, especially your knees and ankles. They can also take up a lot of space and tend to be noisier than other home pieces of equipment. Even a good treadmill changes the way your body would move compared to walking on firm ground, so it's unsuitable for anyone with musculoskeletal injury or pelvic floor weakness. Our advice is to use the ground and trails where you live instead of a treadmill.

Jump rope

Pros: it is cheap and portable and burns a large amount of calories in a short time if you can actually jump rope. Even practicing jump rope can be part of a good warmup to your strength training, so try practicing this for a few minutes before a workout until you get good at this.

Cons: in order to have a training effect from jump roping, you need to have good jumping skills, which may take time to develop. It can be hard on ankles and lower back if you are not in good shape or weigh much more than your optimal weight.

Body weight circuits

Pros: these are a combination of bodyweight exercises, jumping, running and doing specific drills that you can do almost anywhere. They burn a lot of calories and can elevate metabolism for up to two days after a workout. They take a very short time and are very effective.

Cons: you need to know the drills and exercises required by the circuits and be able to do them with good form.

Strength circuits/complexes

Pros: strength circuits and complexes are a step up from bodyweight circuits. You use progressive weight or reps or shorter rest intervals to make these workouts more demanding and effective. They take a very short time and are very effective.

Cons: you need to have great form in a variety of free weight exercises.

Different types of conditioning are suitable during different times of your fat loss program. You don't use a saw mill to cut a strip of molding, do you? We want to use the simplest and easiest to use tools when we start, then progress in complexity and intensity as the program evolves so we never fully adapt to the workouts. If you pull out your best tricks in the beginning, you have little room for improvement. Starting with the easiest exercise first is a key to success. You can always add more later.

Strive for balance

Many people exercise more to make fat loss faster. While this may work for a couple of weeks, over time more exercise can increase your appetite and make it really hard to stick to a sensible style of eating. Always strive for balance and note when you have started moving too much and struggle to maintain your eating plan. If you suspect that your workouts are too strenuous and might be making you fail your diet, you can cut down on the conditioning and just stick to your strength workouts.

Kickstart and Phase 1 Conditioning Options

Earlier, I gave you the option to do one or more days of conditioning during the Kickstart and Phase 1 of your strength training. You can choose to do 1 or more days of any aerobic activity of low to medium intensity. This will not only aid in recovery from the new strength workouts that you are putting yourself through, but it will also help you burn some extra calories. Choose from any of the options below for 30-40 minutes 1-3 times per week.

Walking Fast Uphill – Of course if you have no hill close to you, you could walk fast anywhere, but walking up is a great option. If you have a treadmill, you can easily bump up the incline and use that instead.

Stairs – If you live close to a track or a school, you may have access to bleachers, a nearby park or beach might have stairs, too. Don't forget that office buildings and apartments also have stairs. Climbing stairs burns a lot of calories, so you can do that for about 20 minutes and then walk for an extra 10-15 minutes. If there are no actual stairs, you can try the stairclimber at the gym. We've found the best ones to be setup like an escalator, where the steps move down and you try to keep up.

Stationary Bike/Mountain or Road Bike – Set your bike at an intensity that allows you to carry on a conversation or read, or just head outside and enjoy a 30-40 minute ride on the trail, path, or road.

Phase 2 Conditioning Options

You can now bump up the intensity on your conditioning activities. Take any of the conditioning activities that you have been doing and make them harder by doing bursts of higher intensity work.

If you are particularly heavy, I don't recommend jogging, due to the stress on the joints, so consider starting with our walking option, below. If you have been walking, and feel like you need to step it up a bit, you can now start doing a minute of running and then drop back to walking, if you've been running you can add sprints, etc. Below are examples of how you can structure your workouts, from easier to harder, so that they can include higher intensity intervals.

Walking intervals

5 minutes walking

2 minutes walking as fast as you can walk

2 minutes of slow walking

Repeat 5 times

5 minutes of walking to cool down

This is a total of 30 minutes

Walk/run intervals

5 minutes slow jogging or walking

30 second moderate running

90 second jog/walk

Repeat 5-8 times

5 minutes of jogging to cool down

This will take 20-26 minutes

Sprint intervals

5 minutes jogging

30 second sprint

90 second jog/walk

Repeat 5-8 times

5 minutes of jogging to cool down

This will take 20-26 minutes

Biking intervals

5 minutes leisurely biking

30 second maximum speed pedaling (+ increased resistance)

90 seconds slower biking

Repeat 5-8 times

5 minutes of slow biking to cool down

This will take 20-26 minutes

You can use similar protocols for a rowing machine, an elliptical, a jump rope or any other tool that you have available to you.

Bodyweight Intervals for Phase II

Consider doing bodyweight intervals if none of the options above appeal to you, or use them just to challenge yourself. Bodyweight intervals are fun and will definitely make you feel good about how much fitter you are.

Do the suggested repetitions as fast as possible with good form, doing all the exercises in a row and then taking a 2 minute break (walk around during the break).

Pushups – 5

Reverse lunges – 5 per leg

Mountain climbers – 10 per leg

Bodyweight squats – 5

Wall slides – 10

Repeat 4-6 times

This will take 24-36 minutes

You can substitute any exercise that you like; it's very hard to go wrong on bodyweight intervals.

Phase 3 Conditioning Options.

You can choose to keep doing the interval workouts from Phase II, and just change the duration of the intervals and the rest in between, to make it more challenging. If you were walking in phase 1 and 2, you should be able to run now, although heavier guys can still get a huge benefit from walking and walking intervals.

Jogging

5 minutes jogging

30 second sprint

60 second jog/walk

Repeat 6-8 times

5 minutes of jogging to cool down

This will take 18-22 minutes

Biking

5 minutes leisurely biking

30 second maximum speed pedaling (+ increased resistance)

60 seconds slower biking

Repeat 6-8 times

5 minutes of slow biking to cool down

This will take 18-22 minutes

You can use similar protocols for a rowing machine, an elliptical, a jump rope or any other tool that you have available to you.

Bodyweight Complexes

Of course, bodyweight complexes remain a great option for you, so go ahead and give these a try. Do the suggested repetitions as fast as possible with good form, doing all the exercises in a row and then taking a 1 minute break (walk around during the break).

Jump squats – 5

Pushups – 5

Walking lunges – 5 per leg (walk out and back)

Jumping jacks – 10

Face the wall Ys – 10

Repeat 4-6 times

This will take 24-36 minutes

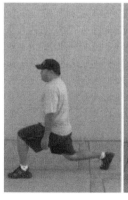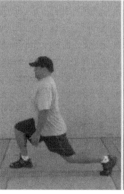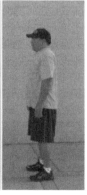

Walking Lunges: Take a step and perform a lunge. Stand up and take a step forward with the trailing leg to lunge again. Continue lunging forward for your total number of reps.

Jump Squats: These are done like regular bodyweight squats, but once you get to the bottom position you will spring up, jump, and gently land down into a bottom squat position. Repeat for all reps.

Weight Complexes

Another option is to do free weight complexes. There are few very *bad* combinations of free weight exercises that you could use for strength complexes, so feel free to improvise. Here is one complex that we have found effective and fun.

Pick a weight that you can overhead press 10 times and do the following exercises in a circuit:

Swings – 10

Goblet Squats – 10

Dumbbell Rows – 10 (5 each side)

One Arm Shoulder Presses – 10 (5 each side)

Suitcase Deadlifts – 10 (5 each side)

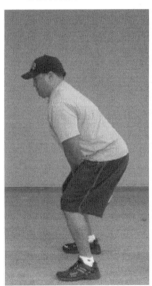
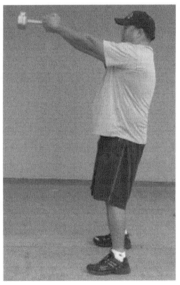

Swings: Stand with your feet wide apart and a dumbbell in your hands. Hinge at the hips, swinging the dumbbell between your legs like you are hiking a football. Powerfully thrust your hips forward to propel the dumbbell up to eye level using just the momentum you generated with your hips. Do not pull with your arms; rather think of them as a rope connecting your body to the weight. Allow the dumbbell to swing back down and through your legs, hinging at the hips to continue with your next swing. Repeat for all reps.

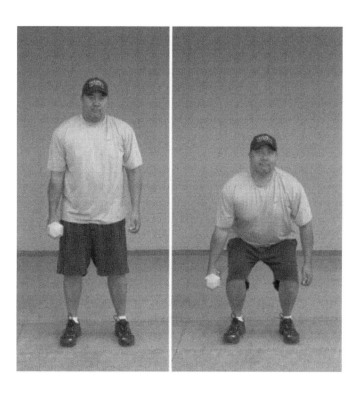

Suitcase Deadlifts: Stand holding one dumbbell at your side. Sit back and down as far as you can without rounding your lower back. Use your glutes to return to the starting position and repeat for all reps on one side, then switch.

Options for taking the workout outside

Say you are in the mood to do something outside. It is perfectly ok not to do your strength workout inside, if you can do something at the playground, the bars at the beach, sun or snow. Outside workouts will charge you with amazing energy and add an extra element of challenge as you do something you are not accustomed to.

What about the playground?

Take your workouts out to the playground by doing a few sets of 5-10 reps of any of the following exercises. New exercises are in **bold**.

Lunges

Bodyweight squats

Pushups

Front planks

Side planks

Jumping jacks –To get more of a sweat, shoot for 15-30 jumping jacks per round.

Pull ups (overhand or straight grip) – When I refer to pullups, I am referring to an overhand grip. You can also do them with palms facing up (chinups) if you like.

167

Squat jumps – this is merely a bodyweight squat, but after you lower yourself down, come up as fast as you can, jumping in the air. Land and immediately squat back down and repeat.

Inverted rows – Pictured below, an Inverted Row is like a pullup, but instead of pulling from the overhead position, your arms are outstretched in front of you. These are not as hard as pullups or chinups, but you have to find a bar low enough.

Mountain climbers – Pictured below, this is just like the Mountain Climbers with Hold from earlier, but do them fast, instead.

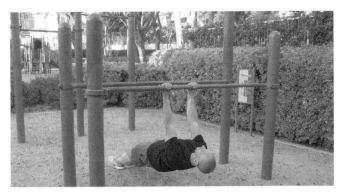

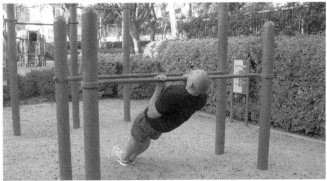

Inverted Rows: Find a low bar in a playground, or even a safety railing, like pictured above. Grab the bar overhand or underhand. Stretch your legs out and straighten your body. Starting with arms outstretched, pull your body up until the bar touches your chest. Lower yourself back down and repeat.

Mountain Climbers – This is just like the Mountain Climbers with Hold from earlier, but do them fast, instead. Alternating legs, bring each leg up to the chest and return to the starting position as fast as possible. Do 5-10 reps before moving on to another exercise.

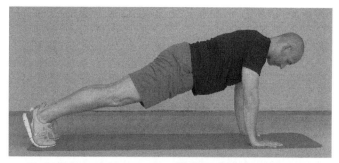

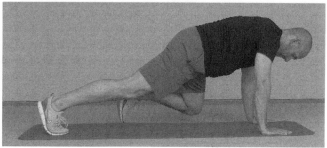

What about the beach?

You might need to save pullups for another day, but you can do these moves, and more! New exercises are in **bold**.

Pushups

Squats, Jump Squats, Lunges, and Walking Lunges

Windshield wipers, Burpees, Sand sprints, and **Bear Crawls**

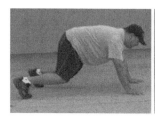 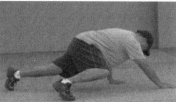

Bear Crawl: These are simply an animal-style crawl, without your knees touching the ground. Get on all fours and lift your hips and knees off the ground. Step forward with you right hand and right foot and crawl forward. Crawl to a point that's 10-20 "crawls" away, then turn around and crawl, walk, or sprint back to the starting point.

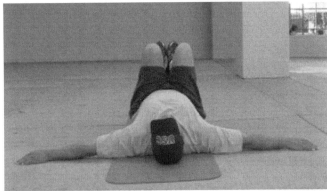

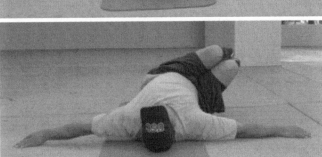

Windshield Wipers: Lie on the ground with your arms stretched out and knees bent to 90 degrees. Lower them to one side. Use your abs to return them to the starting position. Alternate left and right for all reps.

Burpee (no pushup): From a standing position squat down, drop your hands to the ground and jump your feet back to assume a pushup position. Jump your legs forward to between your hands then stand up, raising your arms up into the air. Repeat 5-10 times.

Advanced option 1: Instead of just standing up, jump up, bringing you knees to your chest and your hands into the air over your head. This is the typical burpee, as described in books and on the internet.

Advanced option 2: Do a pushup before jumping your legs forward.

Super Advanced option 3: Do the pushup AND the jump.

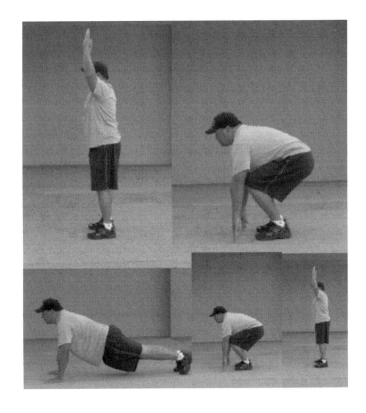

What about the snow?

The snow seems to make everything harder, doesn't it? Don't make the mistake of going heavy with the snow shovel, here. Lighter is better because it means faster shoveling and more calories burned!

Snow shoveling (use one of the smaller shovels and just shovel faster)

High knee walking in deep snow

Pull weights or your kids in a heavy sled

Push weights or your kids in a heavy sled (even harder than pulling)

As you can see, you can literally do your workouts anywhere, at home, outside, on the road, at hotels. Once you know that your body and your weights are your portable gym, you have all the power to lose fat and increase your metabolism. As one of our favorite coaches, Ross Enamait points out, with your body at the ready, "you are never gymless"

What about toys?

TRXs and other suspension trainers, elastic bands, kettlebells, sleds, sledgehammers and tires, sandbags, Bulgarian bags, Power Wheels, battling ropes, clubbells, ab wheels, and gymnastic rings are just some of the hundreds of toys on the market that can add both intensity and variety to your workouts. I certainly recommend adding one or more of them to your workouts if you wish. Galya and I own many of these toys, our friends have most of them, and love to play with them all.

For the purpose of this transformation program, I wanted to keep your equipment and time needs minimal. After all, the point is to make exercise accessible as an option so it can be a lasting part of your life. It's not about fancy toys and equipment, although those things can make it even more fun. This program is about fitting some smart exercise into your weekly routine and doing it in a way that you can maintain for a long time.

11

A day in the life

"

From the movie, Groundhog Day

"What would you do if you were stuck in one place and every day was exactly the same, and nothing that you did mattered?" – Phil Connors

"That about sums it up for me." – Ralph

"

Most guys live a life of patterns, where each day is pretty much the same. Bill Murray's movie, Groundhog Day, was popular because we could all see ourselves in the movie's repetitiveness, even if we didn't get the chance to start each day over again tomorrow.

A repetitive life can be both good and bad, depending on what you do with it. We saw this in Groundhog Day, as well. At first, Phil Connors, Bill Murray's character, spent his repeated days wasting his time and opportunities (including some *very* poor breakfast choices!).

Later in the movie, Bill Murray's character began to use the repetitiveness to his advantage, learning from each day's mistakes or lessons, using the patterns to improve his situation, even though he knew that each day was going to be basically the same day. He finally settled into a perfect rhythm that was smooth and efficient and ideal for achieving his goals. Couldn't you be a real life Phil Connors, using your own Groundhog Days to *your* advantage?

Groundhog Day(s)

Let's take a look and see just how repetitive the typical man's days are. Starting just after waking up, many guys eat breakfast alone, often before the rest of the family even wakes up. Many other guys head off to work and grab something on the road. Some just skip breakfast entirely.

Lunch is usually the same, but different; fast food or a restaurant every day, even if it's a burger one day and tacos the next.

In between breakfast and lunch is any number of snacks, but snack they do; it's often a donut or bagel from the meeting table, but might just as easily be a bag of *miscellaneous* from the vending machine.

Soon, it's dinner time, which is either something his wife made or something he picked up in a drive through on the way home.

Finally, there's dessert or a salty snack. Hopefully not both.

It might be a slightly different pattern for each man, but for each man, each day is pretty much the same pattern. Now that we recognize that there is a pattern, we can try to manipulate it to our advantage. Again, let's start with breakfast.

Breakfast

For many of you, breakfast is "on your own." I get up early and eat before the gym, and in the summer the kids are still snoozing when I'm off to work. I eat alone.

This might sound sad, yes, but it makes my dieting life easy, and you can reap these same benefits. Eat what *you* want or need to eat, not what the family wants to eat; they're still sleeping.

Lunch

If you're like most guys, away from home, on the road, or in the office, lunch is your domain. So dominate it. Here are a few ideas.

Are you eating out with coworkers? – You pick the place as often as possible. It doesn't have to be the healthiest spot, it just needs to have foods that you can handle easily. In my experience, my group spent a lot of time not really knowing where to go, anyway. So, take advantage and make the pick or suggestion for the group. Don't monopolize it, but lead the charge when you can.

Can you pack a lunch? – Childhood picnics got me used to cold chicken, Tupperware veggies, fresh fruit, and plastic forks. You can always go back to that stuff. Also, anything leftover is fair game, and if you have a microwave or kitchenette at the office, all the better.

Galya and I, along with our friend Lisa Wolfe, have a website called Mealsurvivor.com, which has plenty of office ready ideas that are easy to pack or just keep at the office, meaning your diet stays on track, too.

Lunch at home is often one meal where it's every man, woman, and child for himself. That's good news because you can eat what you want, the bad news is that you might have to make two, three, or four different things if you have little kids.

Dinner

Master the meals you can, often breakfast and lunch, and minimize the damage of the others. Dinner is one meal where you often have to eat what's served. By the time you get home, dinner might even be on the table, and there's no telling what's in there. And worse, if you suspect that it's a calorie bomb, what's going to happen if you try to resist eating it?

Our suggestion is to start taking control of dinner whenever you can. The best way to do this is to start cooking. In the next chapter you're going to learn how, using extremely simple recipes that are designed to be healthy, quick, and family friendly. I suggest that you start off slowly, picking one night a week. Master one meal a week, and then experiment with adding more.

You don't need to take over, but the more meals you make, the more you control what goes into your mouth.

I realize that making every dinner isn't the best solution. Your wife is likely a good cook and enjoys cooking, so let her. Just cook when you can and when it works well for the family. You will start to enjoy it more and more, and your wife and family will start to appreciate the new you.

In the next section, "Hunger games," I share tips and tricks to manage those dinners that you can't easily control, minimizing the calorie load, while keeping your cooking and eating relationships as healthy as your new diet.

Snacks

The cultures around the world that don't do much snacking tend to be thinner and fitter than those who seek out the snacks. I recommend that you wean yourself off snacking as much as possible, and just make sure your meals are satisfying enough to get you to your next one.

However, snacks are fully in your control, so keep a stash of healthy snacks in the office, car, or laptop bag.

Dessert

Just like snacking, a regular stream of desserts is a recipe for obesity. My parents grew up with fruit for dessert, unless it was a special occasion. Galya's parents grew up with dessert on Saturday nights and holidays.

Dessert tends to be an after dinner thing, so try to be full and pass on dessert. If you really want something sweet, there's always fruit. When all else fails, keep it small and tasty, and don't waste calories on something that's not delicious.

Control what you can and manage the rest

As your days "repeat," you will learn how to best control what meals you can, while figuring out the best ways to manage the rest. For most people, controlling breakfast, lunch, and snacks, while keeping desserts to a minimum, is a great start. From there, look at dinner, and consider starting to do some cooking for the family.

When cooking dinner isn't an easy option, do your best to manage what you are served. Check out the following section for some great ways to manage those dinners and more.

Hunger games

It's time to cover a few common dilemmas and problems, and the tips and tricks that I recommend for those times. These strategies will help you to more easily manage these situations and events in your life so you can better achieve your weight loss goals in a timely manner.

It's breakfast time, you're hungry, but you don't feel like cooking

Have your coffee or tea, plus water, since you need to get properly hydrated first thing in the morning. You can choose foods that do not require cooking, such as a few pieces of cheese, cold cuts, leftover meat, hard boiled eggs, and a piece of fruit.

You could make a quick protein shake, throwing in a banana, some nuts, seeds, or oatmeal, making it more of a real meal. You could have a protein bar, if a bar is satisfying and filling for you.

You slept in and have no time to eat

You have no time to cook and no time for a shake, but if you skip it, you'll be hungry until lunch. The best strategy is to grab a premade shake or meal replacement from your fridge, or a protein bar or a bag of nuts. If times like this occur often, you may want to keep a stash of protein bars and raw nuts in your car.

Our Cookbook chapter has a recipe for "portable omelets" made in muffin cups. Make some ahead of time and keep them in the fridge for just such an occasion.

The snacks at work, they call to me...

Yeah, they call to me, too.

What, you don't want to succumb to those donuts, cookies, and vending machine treats? Good for you, but when everyone else is munching, you will eventually be tempted, too. It's been shown that if you don't see the snacks you are less likely to eat them. In fact, a fun study showed that secretaries were more likely to eat candy from bowls that were see-through, than those that were opaque. Keep the snacks at bay.

I get so hungry that I don't stop eating until I'm stuffed

This is all too common, as it takes fifteen to twenty minutes for our brains to catch up to our stomachs. Eat too fast and you'll be wishing you wore your special eating pants from Thanksgiving. Come on, you know you have some loose pants, just for those special occasions...

If this is a regular occurrence, try to...

- chew your food longer. I suggest 30 chews per mouthful. More than that and people start to stare.
- put your utensils down between every bite, and don't pick them up again until you've swallowed.
- stop eating when you are 80% full. Wait for 10-15 minutes to see if you're still hungry.

Every desk at work has brownies, candy, and other treats

It's cruel of them, isn't it?

To make sure you can snack healthily when you need to; keep some nuts, jerky, fruit or precut vegetables in your work space.

Divert your attention away from high calorie foods by having coffee or tea, instead. When having coffee, you should watch out for the things you add to your cup, especially sugars and non-dairy creamer. Use only milk or small amounts of half and half in your coffee or tea. Use as little sugar or sweetener as possible, and slowly wean yourself off of them.

Meeting foods are never good choices.

If you have to sit in a meeting with bagels, cookies, or donuts, remember that genetically you are primed to reach for a food when it's available, whether you ate breakfast or not. Since the visual stimulation will make you want to reach for it over and over again, sit far away from it and tell the room that you won't be eating it, right off the bat.

Remind yourself that this is no time for snacking, and that lunch is coming up soon. Realistically, there's no way you're going to subtract those donuts from what you allow yourself to eat at lunch.

If you do cave and eat it, just recognize the mistake and put it behind you. Every meal (or even just a bad food) stands alone. You can get back on track by making your next meal the bare necessities: protein and veggies. You just had plenty of carbs and fat with no nutritional value, so you don't need more of that at lunch.

Every meal stands alone

Resist the urge to throw your diet success out the window because you screwed up once! You didn't screw up the whole day, just the one meal!

It's almost lunch time and you are absolutely "starving."

If you are regularly unable to make it to lunch, add a good breakfast or a small snack to your day. It will be enough to keep you from "starving."

All guys are different – some may have a controlled appetite after fasting all morning. Others might devour their colleague's lunches, in addition to their own; if you're *that* guy, don't skip breakfast again.

You've made it to lunch, but you want to eat the whole menu

For that lunch, have a salad first, or a brothy soup (there's no telling what's in the creamed ones), and then follow with a main dish that's rich in vegetables and protein. If you're going to have some carbohydrate, like a baked potato or a bowl of fruit, don't overeat it.

I need to eat veggies, but salads are a turn off for me

Vegetables, and fruit, do wonders for digestion, fullness and a little something called pH balance that positively influences your general health.

Everyone likes a specific veggie or fruit, so start with those, first. If you don't really like fruit, and you're trying to lose weight, now might not be the right time to add new fruits into your diet, anyway. Focus on adding just one new vegetable each week, whether it's raw or cooked. Maybe you would like grilled vegetables or vegetables in a soup?

Look at the options you have for lunch. If you are bringing your own lunch, you can always bring a fruit or veggie that you like. If you absolutely cannot have vegetables or fruit, you might want to consider a powdered green supplement, such as Greens +.

I eat with my friends, but I'm embarrassed to order "diet food"

You're not ordering cottage cheese and tomato slices are you? Are you are concerned that they will make jokes about your "hold the fries," requests and want to make you eat the same bad stuff they eat? Maybe they need to get in shape, too, but would rather tease you than support you.

It's hard to not have a "get-in-shape team" around you. You may want to just break it to them that you are on a weight loss plan. This way, some of them may join and others may still think you are weird, but doing something for your health should be something to make you proud, not embarrassed.

Are you hungry enough to eat an apple?

There are times when we just want to eat. We may or may not be truly hungry.

"Eat when you are hungry, not when you are bored. If you're not hungry enough to eat an apple, then you're not hungry," says Michael Pollan, author of Food Rules: an Eater's Manual.

I love sandwiches, but I don't know how to make them healthy

To pimp up a sandwich, choose bread like Ezekiel, and thinner slices of rye or whole wheat. On the store shelves, you will see breads called "rounds" and "flats" of 100 calories each. There's no magic to 100 calories, but 100 calories is typically far fewer calories than you would eat if you made a sandwich with regular bread.

Fill it with lean meat, cheese and as many veggies as the bread can hold. Shy away from fillings that have mayo, or heavy sauce, but go for plenty of mustard. On the side, get a fruit bowl or veggies, and hold the chips. While fat free and "baked" chips are certainly a gimmick, there's no denying that they have far fewer calories than their regular versions. If you find them tasty (I do), then choose these over regular chips, and stick to the small, individual serving bags, which are self-limiting.

I get very hungry every day at 4pm

It is pretty common to be hungry at that time, and you don't have to cave into the vending machine junk food or candy dishes near the front desk.

Remember that you can use your own snacks, such as nuts, protein bars or fruit. If you had enough rest the day before and plenty of protein for lunch, you should not be experiencing crazy afternoon munchies that you can't fight off. Should you choose to snack, know that the sweeter the food that you use to satisfy this hunger, the more likely you are to have blood sugar crashes later, making this a snacking rollercoaster.

OMG I want to eat that!

Our good friend Chris Bathke, who's a successful trainer, coach and fat loss mentor to many, wants to eat that thing, too! Man, we all do, but when we have a goal to lose weight, we have to push these things away more often than not.

Chris has his clients ask themselves this question: "does this food or drink take me closer or further from my goal?"

Yeah, review your goals. If you need to, go back and look at your goals from Chapter Three. If that's not enough, stick your goal worksheet to your fridge, where you can see it every day.

What's a good snack to tide me over?

Water, coffee, and tea are good to start, but may simply be unsatisfying for some people. Solid food snacks include hardboiled eggs, string cheese, nuts, a small apple or banana, raw veggies, jerky, and a small protein bar.

Don't choose a snack based on how much you like it, instead, choose a snack based on how well it satisfies you and keeps you there until your next scheduled meal.

The pre-meal ritual

Sometimes I get really hungry before dinner time...

It's natural for the sounds and smells of dinner to get your digestive juices flowing well before it's time to eat. Unfortunately, it can lead to overeating when dinner comes. A "tide me over" snack often just whets the appetite, and you end up eating that AND the large dinner; it's the rare man who reduces his meal size to make up for the pre-meal snack.

Strangely, eating something small before a main meal has actually been shown to minimize the calories you will eat at the big meal coming up, provided you do things right. You can't just have any old snack and hope for the best.

Gal and I call it our "pre-meal strategy," or the de-appetizer, and it's based on studies and experiments which looked at various pre-meal foods and the effect that they had on the size of the meal that followed.

What the studies and experiments found was that an apple, a small bowl of soup, or a modest salad, eaten 15 minutes prior to the meal caused diners to eat 150 to 200 calories less than they would have eaten had they not had the snack. Those calories include the calories of the pre-meal food, so you're coming out ahead.

Pre-meal foods, or the "de-appetizer"

• A ½ can of soup. Creamy and blended soups seems to work better than brothy, but remember to keep it under 150 calories.

• 1 oz of cheese – this is pretty small, so serve with a small plate of veggies.

• 2 hardboiled eggs – You can even try deviled eggs, but avoid the high calorie mayo and use mustard only.

• 2-3 cups of salad – go easy on the dressing, and make sure it comes in under 150 calories. You can also look at the chopped salads in the Cookbook section, as they tend to be more filling and satisfying than a salad of lettuce, and require less dressing to be delicious.

• Keep them at 150 calories or less – just enough to register, not enough to fill you up.

• Make it part of the family meal. A small salad, a plate of vegetables (called a relish tray in the olden days), or a cup of soup works well.

• At the meal, don't load up your plate, instead serve yourself less, and then go back if you really need more.

My wife's food is too good

Yes, and she's too good looking, her breasts are too large, and she's always all over you. You poor man.

Does your wife cook delicious meals, but with so many calories, you feel like you should just skip dinner? Lasagna, spaghetti, and tuna casseroles can be calorie bombs. Not only are they terribly tasty, but they are filled with delicious calories, then jammed into tiny little servings that are horribly unsatisfying. Who can eat just one square of lasagna?

First, I hope you've already had that conversation with your wife and assured her that her food is delicious, but you just can't eat as much as you'd like to right now. Maybe she can save some of the more calorie rich favorites for special occasions.

Second, I hope you've tried the "pre-meal ritual" that I just covered in the previous sidebar. After some soup or a "de-appetizer," your eyes won't be bigger than your appetite should be.

Third... Take your standard dinner plate; it's a big one. Now, put it back and get a smaller one. Good boy. Smaller plates make smaller portions look bigger and more satisfying. Don't get ridiculous and use a saucer; just don't use a huge plate. If you only have really big sized or saucer sized, you might need to buy some in-between ones.

Fourth. Let's hope your wife loves you and understands you and your goals here. If she does, she probably has some sort of salad or low calorie vegetables on the table. If she doesn't, then consider keeping salad greens or prepared or raw veggies around for these occasions. However you get it, put a lot of this stuff on your plate. Loading up your plate with low calorie foods is one way of limiting the high calorie foods, but still giving you enough physical food to fill your belly.

Fifth. Take some of the main dish, but not all you want. Here's where you have to use some judgment. You can't take as much as you really want, because you really want more than you need. That's why you're reading this book, right?

When I was getting smaller, one thing that I did was watch the amounts of food that my skinny friends ate, and then only eat about as much as they did. You can try that here. Assuming your wife eats a smaller amount than you do, eat the same portion that she does. You have to be smart about it – if she's only eating the lasagna and no veggies, it may be too big. If she's always eaten the same size servings as you, it may be too big. If she's overweight, it may be too big. And so on.

Most people know how much they should eat, they just eat too much anyway, especially when it's delicious. It's annoying to eat the right amount of lasagna, isn't it? The right amount of lasagna is too little to be satisfying. Suck it up and remember that you have a plate full of other things. Plus, this is only one meal. You can be more satisfied tomorrow.

Food is fuel (or life isn't fair)

It really isn't fair. I can't have all the burgers I want and stay lean. You can't have two squares of lasagna and lose weight. For most of us, dessert every night is a recipe for getting fat.

Food wasn't always delicious, you know. Once, food was just fuel for our bodies. Then, spices, deep frying, fondue forks, and ranch dressing came along. They came and they changed the game. Now, we expect food to be tasty. We, of course, "deserve" to be able to have food we love and be fully satisfied. But, sometimes we have to choose moderation to get or stay slim and healthy. In these cases, larger amounts of lower calorie foods can be more satisfying than smaller amounts of extremely tasty dishes.

If it helps, get in the mindset of other people who have been hungry, like a monk for instance. Not the Friar Tuck sort of monk; he was sort of tubby. More like the Kwai Chang Caine (from 70s television show 'Kung Fu') type of monk. Caine trekked across the old west, living a Spartan existence, eating fuel, not meals. He searched for somebody or something – the one armed man or The Hulk, I think. I don't really remember – but he wasn't concerned about the satisfaction of his meals, he was concerned about the energy to keep searching.

Soldiers can be hungry, too. On the march, in a plane, in a tank; they eat what they can. Rations are fuel, and are designed to be "edible," not fine dining.

"Food is fuel. Continue the march" - Captain Dale Dye, USMC

If you think about it, our bodies don't make us fat, our minds do. Our bodies need the energy to move and live, while our minds crave taste, comfort, and pleasure, leading us to eat more than we need, essentially over-fueling our bodies.

If you need to, just eat and move on. Fuel up just enough, then use that fuel as you're supposed to. Be that monk. Be that soldier.

Conquer, don't cave

In this chapter I covered the daily life of modern man, and I left you with a few important strategies to use for when you've done everything right, but *you're just damned hungry!*

Follow the six healthy diet tenets, keep reading labels, focus on the good guys and avoid the bad guys, and when you're hungry, get yourself in the mindset to conquer rather than cave!

The healthy diet tenets

The evidence seems to point out that sensible calories, the right fats, the right amount of protein, the inclusion of vegetables and fruits, and a decent activity level are what it takes to make a diet healthy.

1. Calories – only as many as you need.

2. Fats – avoid the bad and look for the good.

3. Veggies – vegetables are full of fiber and nutrients... eat up!

4. Protein – muscle building and filling.

5. Fruits – it's what's for dessert.

6. Activity – either hunt and gather for the first 5 tenets or head outside to play.

Success in the spotlight #4

Cataract surgery left him unable to exercise

After cataract surgery, doctors told him he would not be able to exercise. At all.

Overweight and out of shape at the age of 24, Spas was determined to find an answer. By coming to train with Galya, Spas was able to find an approach that worked around his physical limitations. Now, 5 years later, he is sporting a body closer to his ideal of fitness and health than ever before!

Spas Smilenov, 29 years old and 20 pounds lighter at 168 pounds

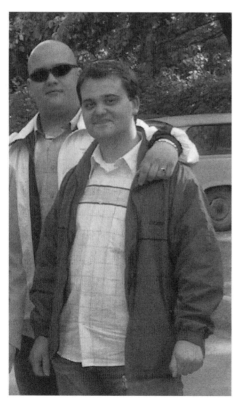

Spas, before, with his brother

Galya – How old were you when you started losing weight and getting fit?

Spas – 25 years old

Galya – Do you know what was wrong with your diet when you started?

Spas – Yes, I was only eating at night. I wasn't sleeping enough. I was having a lot of sodas, chocolate, and too much rice and potatoes.

Galya – How did you train to achieve your results?

Spas – Hard and regular. I followed the advice of my mentors, like you. And never ever said "It's too hard for me!"

Galya – Did your training change with time?

Spas – Yes, I have been adding more and new types of exercises, because my goal is to see a six pack. I am not at the finish line yet, but I am closer than ever.

Galya – I know it wasn't easy for you to start. What were your limiting factors?

Spas – I had just had eye surgery. They told me not to do *any* physical activity. No weights, no running, no jumping. Nothing heavier than an empty jar. I had just graduated from Architecture school in 2007, and I was very weak, I had no muscle or energy after 6 years of just drawing night and day. I decided to make a change and found you on the Internet, and joined your gym.

Spas – You were the only person who would work with me, my doctor, and my eye problems. Starting slowly was the key. That was the beginning of a miracle that lasts to this day for me. Training has given me a new look and my new life!

Galya – Did you have friends that supported you? Did your family support you?

Spas – Actually my family supported me, but not all of my friends supported me. They said that I was too old for this. Those people are crabs, they just want to bring you down, so I try not to hear them.

Galya – What do you think made you gain weight before?

Spas – I think I was eating just too many sweets, too much cheese, and I wasn't moving enough.

Galya – What are your strategies for managing your diet at work?

Spas – For me it's important that I always think about my goal and I pursue it ! I always think about that when choosing my food.

Galya – What about when you have to spend a long time with relatives, what are your strategies?

Spas – That is always difficult. I try to drink more water, and try to sample everything at the table, but in very small amounts.

Galya – What are your strategies to reduce the damage of any big meals?

Spas – After big meals my tip is to take a walk. Moving also allows me to vent the frustration I feel if I overeat – it's easy to not like yourself when you have binged. Walking it off helps me to take care of that, and I start fresh when I come back.

Galya – You have been making amazing progress for many years, what motivates you?

Spas – To me, it's been very, very important to look good and to feel younger, so that keeps me going. The mirror is right there.

Galya – Do you have any tips for people who get frustrated with dieting and training?

Spas – Yes, one! Be patient, and always follow the diet, the training, and the plan; do not stop! It's not important to lose *fast*. It is more important to be cool and fun and succeed, long term, and then remember to see the true man that you are in your mirror. :-)

Galya – Do you have favorite resources that inspire you?

Spas – People inspire me or motivate me – Yordan Yovchev, Hugh Jackman, Cam Gigandet, for instance.

Galya – Sure. Do you think it's easier for people to eat and train well in Bulgaria than it is in the United States?

Spas – Yes, I think so. Here, we have more natural foods. But many people are challenged by things like hamburgers from all the new fast food restaurants. These foods can attract people a lot more than our normal foods can, and that's a big problem.

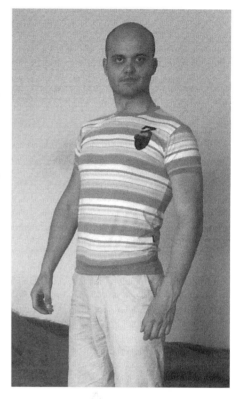

Spas Smilenov is an architect in Bulgaria.

Juggling a professional career as an architect and entrepreneur with very little free time, Spas finds a way to train everywhere - in a gym, at home, on the road, and has his eyes set on his goal - to improve and improve beyond his imagination.

He is always in search of a better training approach, reads voraciously and keeps growing his support network of fitness professionals.

A man with a dream and determination cannot be stopped, and Spas is a living proof of that.

12

Cookbook

A guy's gotta eat, might as well be good

I'm told that I write too much when I should really just net it out. I'm sure this is a prime example. Here I have an opportunity to list a bunch of recipes for you, but instead I'm writing yet another introduction. If all you want is recipes, skip ahead, down to the list (it's labeled "Recipes").

People make cooking hard

It's not.

People have been cooking for a long time – slightly less than 6,000 years according to some and more than 1.8 million years according to others. Most of this time was spent grilling. I don't have a reference for that, but when I once asked my archeologist friend, Dr. John Williams, whether it was mostly grilling, he said "yes."

Grilling is simple, needing only fire, food, and maybe a stick or an actual grill. Yes, we've come a long way since then. By adding spices, rubs, marinades, and Teflon, grilling has become an art, spawning books on the subject that now make even grilling complicated.

I have nothing against complicated recipes, but when they scare a person away from something that's so simple, it is a bit of an issue to me. Authors and publishers seem to agree, judging by the many books that highlight that their recipes only have 5, 4, or even 3 ingredients. It's hard to imagine anything really special in the three ingredient books, but you never know. Many of us have had a perfect backyard steak seasoned with just salt and pepper, or trout fried in butter over a campfire. Depending on how you count, the ingredient list is safely under 5, 4, or even 3. This is good food at its simplest, and there's my point – food can be simple AND good at the same time, and complicating it doesn't necessarily make it better, as many steak purists know.

Most of the meals in this book contain very few ingredients. The foods are good and the ingredients tend to stand alone. There's nothing fundamentally wrong with long ingredient lists, either. They have their place, and there's no arguing that they possess many subtleties that can "take foods to the next level." However, long ingredient lists are confusing and overwhelming, and can easily lead to mistakes, panic, accidents, and often, bad food.

These long lists have long been such a well-known problem to the new cook that television sitcoms and romantic comedy films often use them to create "situations." These usually result in a kitchen covered with flour, blended sauces on the ceiling, a grease fire, a fire extinguisher, and a visit from the fire department. And, as we see on the TV screen, they usually result in giving up and going out for pizza, and a vow never to cook again.

In an earlier chapter, I told you to control what meals you could control, and manage the rest. I showed you the "manage" part, and now it's time to take some control.

Taking control

Taking control sounds ominous, but don't get excited. You're not going to need to dominate anyone, yell, or even lay down the law. All you have to do is start cooking.

When you cook, you choose the ingredients. You know what and how much is in there. Dish it out yourself and you've taken control of your own diet. It's that simple.

If you're like me, you eat totally different breakfasts and lunches than the rest of the family. I don't know where this tradition started, but my kids and I eat different things at these meals. It's a free for all, mostly. Sometimes we sit down to eat a hot breakfast, but most of the time we all open the fridge on our own and get what we want. Lunch and snacks follow the same pattern in my house, and asking around, this seems pretty standard these days. We could discuss if this is the best way to handle family meals, but today we need baby steps, not giant leaps.

Many of the guys I know cook about a meal a week, but only while it's summer and grilling season is upon us. Once the weather turns cold and it gets dark early, no one wants to stand out there flipping meat on the barbeque, so it's back to cooking about zero meals a week. A first baby step could be to start cooking inside, too. It's not as hard or as daunting as it sounds.

You're a guy, and like most guys, you are probably comfortable grilling. It's like an instinct, and mixing fire and meat comes naturally to you. In grilling, even the sides are simple. Some guys boil a bunch of corn on the side burner and some grill veggies right on the grill. The guys that make their own garlic bread have taken things to the next level. This is simple food at its simplest, and surprisingly, the family eats it. They don't question anything or complain. There's very little "this isn't how Mom makes it." They just eat it because it's good and because you cooked it.

Confidence is key. It's way more than half the battle. Why are you confident grilling? Because it's simple and you've done it many times. Some might say it's foolproof, but that's setting the wrong expectations. Grilling isn't foolproof. You have to watch what you're doing and make sure it's not burned or raw, but you know you have leeway either way. It's still going to be good, whether it's a bit more grilled than you like or whether you had to toss it back on the grill for five more minutes to finish cooking through.

Tenets of guy cooking

1 – Real food can be simple and still good

I think "steak" pretty much sums up the concept. Steak is simple and good. Guys are simple. Be simple. Cook simply.

2 – Change the game

Don't make diet lasagna. Don't make diet chocolate cake. Don't take a family favorite and try to make it healthy; that usually just makes it a lesser version of something the family loves. Make something that's new to you and new to the other people eating with you. Want soup? Don't makeover your Mom's matzo ball soup, make a healthy mulligatawny soup. What's mulligatawny? No one knows, so how can you have made a lesser version?

3 – Don't cook the same things your wife cooks, trust me

Just think about these conversations...

"Why would you want to make over my stew?"

"So, you think my lasagna is unhealthy?"

"You don't like tuna casserole?"

"That was my mom's chicken."

"You don't like *my* tuna casserole."

"That was my grandma's meat loaf. "

"You don't like my *mom's* tuna casserole?"

"You think I'm fat."

"My grandma is dead, you know. "

...think about it.

4 – Allow side dishes that aren't part of your meal

Just because you limit your own pasta consumption doesn't mean your skinny family has to. They will revolt if you do.

This doesn't mean you can't make perfectly healthy meals for them, but fill them up with the healthy and allow a little slack on the side. Serve more meat and veggies and smaller portions of rice, for instance.

It helps to pick things that you don't really like. I could care less about cornbread, so if there's a pan of that crap on the table, I'll stick to my chili.

5 – They will eat it because you cooked it

You have a window of opportunity while you "learn what they like" or subconsciously convince them that they like what you're cooking. ...all the while, you learn how to cook.

If you change the game, keep it simple, and allow them the freedom to add what they want to your meal, they will be surprisingly accommodating. Your wife, mother, or girlfriend will (or should) appreciate the break from cooking. Just make sure to clean up after yourself (details on that in the next book).

Once you have a few meals down pat, your family will enjoy them even more, even if your meals are totally different foods than those your wife makes. Make it and they will eat.

Now, on to the food, itself.

Recipes

Be master of your breakfast

Like I talked about in the last chapter, for many guys, weekday breakfasts are "on your own." Of course, the weekends are a different story. You might all eat breakfast together. If so, then control what you can, minimize the calorie bombs, and substitute when it's appropriate.

Of course, you could also be that dad who cooks breakfast – his way—on Saturday or Sunday or even both. See? You're back in control!

Many of our breakfast recipes are fast and easy, so you can get up and out, satisfied and ready to slave away at work. Others are slower paced, and good for when you have more time. I also have a few that can work for the weekends, when you might also be serving breakfast for the family.

Oatmeal

Some people tend to find oatmeal VERY satisfying so this is your chance to see if that works for you. To make perfect oatmeal, you have two options: keep it cold, or make it hot. I offer you recipes for both.

I'm going to assume that you're most likely making breakfast for yourself, most of the time, so the recipes in the breakfast section are primarily written with just one person in mind.

Keep it cool oatmeal

Serves 1

Ingredients

1 cup rolled oats

1 oz almonds

A few drops vanilla extract

½ cup milk

Directions

The night before you plan to eat this, cover oatmeal with cold water, add the almonds and leave in the fridge. In the morning, add the vanilla and milk, stir well and enjoy. If you feel like sweetening the oatmeal, add a tbsp. of honey or maple syrup.

Still hungry: add a few pieces of string cheese (um, on the side...)

Hot apple cinnamon oatmeal

Serves 1

Ingredients

1 cup rolled oats

1 small apple

2 tbsp peanut butter

Cinnamon to taste

Directions

To make, bring 2 cups water to a boil, add the oatmeal, turn the heat to medium and cook for 5 minutes, occasionally stirring. In the meantime, wash and grate an apple, and place in a bowl. Take the oatmeal off the heat, stir in the peanut butter, add the apple and cinnamon and enjoy.

Protein power oatmeal

Serves 1

Ingredients

1 cup rolled oats

1 tbsp butter

1 scoop protein powder

1/2 oz walnuts

Directions

To make the oatmeal, bring 2 cups water to a boil, add the oatmeal, turn the heat to medium and cook for 5 minutes, occasionally stirring. While still hot, add the butter and stir in the protein powder. Vanilla is our favorite, but chocolate works too. Top with 1/2 oz walnuts.

Omelets

I can't give enough praise to a well-cooked omelet - I promise if you like eggs, this can be a breakfast you will never ever tire of.

Despite those who claim that a perfect omelet can be made in cast iron or stainless steel pans, I recommend a good non-stick skillet, which allows you to use less oil and make an omelet that doesn't fall apart and frustrate you.

California omelet

Serves 1

Ingredients

4 eggs

1 tsp oil (ghee, expeller pressed coconut or light olive oil)

Salt and pepper to taste

1 oz cheddar cheese

¼ avocado

4 tbsp salsa

Directions

Whisk the eggs together, but don't overbeat them. In a large nonstick pan, heat up the oil, pour the eggs and cook on both sides. Sprinkle the cheddar on top and fold. Serve on a large plate. Cut up the avocado and place on top. Cover with the salsa. Feel free to serve a cup of cherry tomatoes or carrots along if you feel like you need more volume.

The meat lover's omelet

Serves 1

Ingredients

3 eggs

2 pork links (cooked)

1 oz mozzarella cheese, grated

1 tsp oil (ghee, expeller pressed coconut or light olive oil)

Chili powder

1 green bell pepper

Directions

Whisk the eggs together and cut up the pork links in small chunks. Mix in the mozzarella cheese, grated. Heat up the oil, pour in the mixture and cook on both sides till golden. Fold and serve, sprinkle with chili powder and cut up the bell pepper to enjoy on the side.

Sweet omelet

For those mornings when you have a sweet tooth

Serves 1

Ingredients

3 eggs

2 tbsp heavy cream

4-5 drops vanilla extract

1-2 tbsp raisins

1 tsp oil (ghee, expeller pressed coconut or light olive oil)

1 tbsp honey

2 tbsp cream cheese

Directions

Whisk the eggs, the heavy cream and the vanilla extract. Add the raisins. Heat the oil over medium heat, cook the omelet on both sides till golden. Fold with the cream cheese inside. Garnish with the honey and enjoy. Keep this away from your wife, these have been known to disappear mysteriously.

Frittatas

A cool, and lazier way to make an omelet - bake it. You can do that the night before your breakfast or you can heat up the oven and throw the frittata in there while you take a shower in the morning - I love these so much I urge you to cook more and take the leftovers to work with you.

Spinach and mushroom frittata

Serves 1

Ingredients

3 whole eggs

¼ cup chopped mushrooms

½ cup cooked or thawed, drained spinach

6 olives, pitted, sliced

1 oz grated jack cheese

1 garlic clove, chopped

Pinch salt

Pinch black pepper

Directions

Heat the oven to 400F. Use a fork and a deep bowl to mix the eggs without beating them too much. Gently add the rest of the ingredients and stir them in. Pour everything in a small cast iron pan and cook for 20 min.

Roasted pepper, ham and artichoke frittata

Serves 1

Ingredients

3 whole eggs

¼ cup chopped roasted peppers

½ cup thawed artichoke hearts, chopped

2 oz ham, smoked, cubed

1 oz grated sharp cheddar

1 small green onion, chopped

Pinch salt

Pinch black pepper

Directions

You can get roasted peppers in a jar in the deli section of your store (where you buy the olives). You can also roast them yourself if you have the time.

Heat the oven to 400F. Use a fork and a deep bowl to mix the eggs without beating them too much. Gently add the rest of the ingredients and stir them in. Pour everything in a small cast iron pan and cook for 20 min.

Shakes

Shakes are for those mornings when you are really in a hurry but determined to get your breakfast. They are also great before a workout when you don't feel like eating something heavy. You will need a blender, and a high quality protein powder supplement. Try to find a protein powder that doesn't contain soy, and is dairy (milk, whey and/or casein) or egg based. If you simply don't eat animal products, a plant based supplement is fine, but choose protein sources other than soy, which can be highly estrogenic in men.

Banana shake

For this classic you just need to peel a banana and place it in the freezer.

Serves 1

Ingredients

1 banana, frozen, chunks

1 cup milk

1 scoop protein powder

Dash vanilla extract

Directions

Place everything in the blender and blend until smooth on high. Serve immediately and enjoy.

Coffee shake

This is the perfect pick me up when you are in a hurry to have your breakfast and coffee all in one.

Serves 1

Ingredients

1 cup milk

1 scoop protein powder

Shot espresso

5 ice cubes

Directions

Blend on high until you get a smooth consistency. If you feel like an extra kick, add a double shot of espresso instead.

Wild berry shake

Feeling like a shake that will keep you full longer? Try this:

Serves 1

Ingredients

2/3 cup plain yogurt

1 scoop protein powder

½ frozen mixed berries

1 tbsp honey

Directions

Place all ingredients in the blender and mix well.

Peanut butter and chocolate shake

Being in a hurry doesn't mean you can't indulge in a delicious shake that will rock your taste buds first thing in the morning.

Serves 1

Ingredients

1 ¼ cups milk

1 scoop protein powder

1 tbsp peanut butter

1 tbsp unsweetened cocoa

Directions

Place all ingredients in the blender and mix well. You may need to stop midway and make sure all peanut butter has been mixed in before you pour.

What kinds of milk should I use?

I recommend organic full fat cow's milk, but if you can't have cow's milk, you can have almond, rice, oat, or coconut milk. Soy is very controversial, so I don't recommend it.

Here are your best choices of "milks" in the order that I recommend:

Cow's un-homogenized organic milk

Cow's homogenized organic milk

Goat's organic milk

Coconut milk (canned, but you'll have to thin it with water)

Coconut boxed (in the milk section and already thinned to be more like milk)

Almond milk

Rice milk

Oat milk

Quinoa milk

Hemp Milk

Keep in mind that nearly all of these "milks" have thickeners and gums to make them seem more like the milk that you grew up with. Read the labels and consider that you might be taking in a lot of added sugars and other ingredients just to have "milk." If it's for your shakes, consider protein powder and water instead of milk substitutes; you'll get a big shot of protein and less added sugar in return.

Protein Pancakes

Here is a cool way to enjoy pancakes with a bit of added protein, so you can be a part of the family breakfast or just because you have some extra time one morning. I am suggesting our two favorite kinds, but if you feel like a plain pancake just skip the fruit.

Blueberry pancakes

Even Alan Aragon likes these ;)

Serves 1 (4 pancakes)

Ingredients

3 eggs

1 1/2 scoop protein powder (vanilla is best)

3 tbsp oat bran/wheat bran/rolled oats

A handful of blueberries

1 tsp coconut oil

Directions

Whisk the eggs and protein powder, add the bran, wheat bran or rolled oats (use what you have handy) and at the end carefully fold in the blueberries. Coat the pan with coconut oil over medium heat and spoon in half of the mixture. Flip over when golden brown and repeat for the other pancakes.

Serve with a small amount of honey or maple syrup. If you feel like you need a more generous amount, use light syrup. I personally find that a small amount of jelly or peanut butter is a lot more satisfying than light syrup, which tastes good but makes you hungry again very soon.

Banana pancakes

This is another classic that will make you wish you had started this healthier eating plan sooner.

Serves 1 (4 pancakes)

Ingredients

3 eggs

1 1/2 scoop protein powder (vanilla is best)

2 tbsp pancake mix or flour

2 tbsp milk

1 banana

1 tsp coconut oil

Directions

Mix the eggs, protein, pancake mix and milk. Cut the banana in thin circles. Place the pan over medium heat and coat it with some coconut oil. Pour enough pancake mixture for 1 pancake, give it a few seconds and then arrange a few banana circles flat side down so you have covered the surface of the pancake. Flip over and cook until done.

Smart snacking

There are times when snacks are needed, and when they are, most of our snacks are just like our lunches; leftovers, meat, cheese, hardboiled eggs, fruit, veggies. These might sound boring, but are you hungry or looking for entertainment?

Hardboiled eggs

Makes 12 eggs (3 is typically good for a snack)

Ingredients

12 eggs

Directions

Place eggs in a pan and cover with cold water. Bring to a boil, then cover and turn the heat off. Let the eggs and water sit for about 10 minutes, then drain the water.

Fill a large bowl with ice water. Lightly crack each egg and then put it in the bowl of ice water. After 5-10 minutes, drain, and refill with more cold water and then put the bowl in the refrigerator until the eggs are fully cooled. Drain and peel them all now or store them in something covered until you are ready to use them.

Hint – fresher eggs tend to be harder to peel, so use your older eggs to hard-boil, not your newest ones.

Beef Jerky Trail Mix

Yeah, sounds weird, but it's so good and satisfying. Why eat jerky out of one hand and trail mix out of the other? This is a real time saver.

Your ingredients should be chosen to be satisfying, so don't waste calories on things you don't care about (that would be sunflower seed kernels for me). I use ingredients that make it chewy and crunchy (so it takes work to eat), sweet and salty (so it tastes awesome), and satisfying enough to keep me good until the next feeding time.

For unusual, healthy, and satisfying ingredients, check out the bulk food bins at the local health food store.

Makes 6 servings

Ingredients

4 oz nuts (raw, roasted, salted, or unsalted – your choice)

2 oz pumpkin seeds (dry roasted and still in the shell)

2 oz beef jerky (chopped into small pieces)

1 oz dried apple or apple chips (broken or chopped)

1 oz unsweetened coconut chips or flakes

Directions

Chop it all up, and then stir and shake it together. Measure it into small zipper bags or tiny plastic containers.

Trail mix is a trigger food for me, so I try not to keep too much around the house. If you binge on this stuff, only make as much as you know you should eat and portion it out ahead of time.

Dinner, when it's your turn to cook

Quick, review the tenets of guy cooking, just to refresh your memory.

1 – Real food can be simple and still good

2 – Change the game

3 – Don't cook the same things your wife cooks, trust me

4 – Allow them sides that aren't part of your plan

5 – They will eat it because you cooked it

Comfortable? Good.

Meat, poultry, & fish

If a guy has enough meat, a guy has dinner. For many men, meat is the basis of a meal—walking through an all you can eat buffet, he's looking for the prime rib station or huge pile of crab legs. When arriving at Aunt So and So's for Thanksgiving... "How big's that bird?"

The meat is "where it's at." Everything else is secondary. Meat and potatoes. I rest my case.

Roasted Chicken, Fast!

Serves 4 or more

Roasted chicken is a great dish to have around for leftovers. After you make one, you'll see how versatile it can be for salads, soup, snacks, and lunches. This one is pretty quick to make. Melinda Lee, the host of a great radio cooking show in Los Angeles, has a version of this that she calls "Blasted Chicken." She cautions you on the smoke that can come from the high heat and chicken fat, so I will too; open a window and use the range hood fan.

Ingredients

1 frying or broiling chicken (3-4½ lbs)

Salt and pepper

Directions

Preheat the oven to 450 degrees.

Rinse the chicken and dry it off with paper towels. Salt and pepper the bird pretty good, inside and out. Put the chicken in a shallow roasting pan. Insert a meat thermometer in the thickest part of the thigh, not touching the bone. Roast for 45 minutes (55 if the fryer is over 4 pounds), opening a window a bit, because there might be some smoke! Remove from the oven and let the chicken stand, untouched, for 15 minutes. DO NOT start to cut the chicken until the 15 minutes has passed, got it? Good.

One Dish Tip – Cut up some potatoes, carrots, yams, turnips, etc. and toss them with some coconut oil or leftover bacon fat, salt, and pepper. Scatter them around the chicken. They will absorb a mysterious amount of the chicken fat, and help with the smoking problem. They are delicious, but since the calories are mysterious and the starchy foods may not fit with your goals today, this may be the part your family eats while you take a pass. They are really tasty, so the family may thank you for your sacrifice.

Pan Grilled Chicken Tenderloins or Boneless Breasts

Frozen chicken tenderloins (the tenderloin is merely the best part of the chicken breast with the extras removed) are very convenient. They come in huge bags and are individually quick frozen, so you only use what you need. Even better, you can usually cook them quickly without thawing. The bag should have clear instructions to bake, roast, or pan fry.

Breasts are almost as convenient, but since they are thicker and not always the same size and shape, you may have to thaw them beforehand. To cook them faster and make them look prettier, follow these instructions for flattening the breasts. It's not hard, and it makes cooking them a breeze.

To flatten chicken breasts, put a thawed breast into a heavy duty zipper bag and zip it closed while squeezing all the air out of it. Place it on a heavy cutting board and gently pound it flat with a heavy pan or even a 2x4. They actually make a special tool for this, but it's not necessary.

Now, don't just hammer away, you sort of work from the center on out. Hammer in waves. Repeat with all the chicken breasts. After you've flattened them, trim them down to manageable portions. The goal is to end up with fillets that are all even in thickness and can be cooked and served in manageable sizes.

By the way, you can flatten chicken tenderloins, too. They are even easier, since they start off smaller and thinner.

Ingredients

6-8 oz of chicken breast per person (thawed and flattened, if desired)

Cooking spray or 1 tsp light olive oil

Water or broth

Salt to taste

Directions

Use a large shallow and non-stick skillet here. The pan needs to be large enough for all pieces of chicken to fit at once, or just do it in batches. Lightly spray the non-stick skillet with cooking spray or oil. Heat the pan over medium high heat.

Sprinkle the chicken with a little salt, then add the chicken and cook for about 5 minutes, shaking the pan and moving the chicken pieces to keep them from sticking. Turn the chicken once and then add a little water to the pan. Add just enough to come about halfway up the sides of the chicken. Do not cover the pan.

Simmer for about 15 minutes. The liquid should be reduced by about half, and they should no longer be pink inside if you cut one to test. Salt to taste.

Easy Meatloaf

This makes eight servings, so you might have plenty of leftovers for your lunches.

8 servings

Ingredients

2 lbs lean ground beef

2 eggs

1 tbsp ground cumin

1 teaspoon black pepper

1 teaspoon sea salt

3 tbsp tomato paste or catsup for glazing

Directions

Preheat oven to 400 degrees.

In a large bowl, mix the beef, eggs, spices, salt, and pepper. Mix until well combined. Form into a loaf shape and place on a cookie sheet or baking pan. If possible, let it sit for 30 minutes to an hour before baking.

Bake for 45-60 minutes, then remove the loaf from the oven and glaze it with the tomato paste. Return the loaf to the oven and bake an additional 15 minutes until a meat thermometer registers at least 150 degrees.

Mushroom and Sun Dried Tomato Meatloaf

This makes eight servings, so you might have plenty of leftovers for your lunches.

8 servings

Ingredients

2 lbs lean ground beef

1 cup sun dried tomatoes (dried or in olive oil)

1 tbsp olive oil (you can use some oil from the sundried tomatoes)

1 cup ground up dry mushrooms

2 tbsp oregano

1 teaspoon black pepper

1 teaspoon sea salt

2 eggs

½ cup pitted olives (black, green, or mixed)

3 tbsp tomato paste for glazing

Directions

Coarsely grind the dried mushrooms in a mortar and pestle, food processor, or blender.

If the tomatoes are dried, then they need to be reconstituted. Bring a cup of water to boiling and pour over the sun dried tomatoes. Let them sit for 15-20 minutes and then drain them.

Preheat oven to 425 degrees.

Chop the tomatoes, and add the beef, mushrooms, olive oil, eggs, salt, and spices. Mix well and let it sit for 30 minutes to an hour.

Lay out a large sheet of foil. Form a rectangle of meat on the foil. Spread the olives evenly on top and then roll the meatloaf, grabbing the aluminum foil from the bottom and using it to support the meat. Once rolled, move the meatloaf to a meatloaf pan or baking dish. Using your finger, make three evenly spaced holes along the top of the loaf.

Bake for 45 minutes, then remove the loaf from the oven and glaze it with the tomato paste. Return the loaf to the oven and bake an additional 15 minutes.

Burgers

I used to joke with my friends that I was on a low carb diet, and then I'd order a double cheeseburger instead of my usual two burgers. Half the bread, half the carbs!

After a while, I stopped ordering fries, and pretty soon I was just eating the meat, cheese, and veggies. At this point, I was telling my friends that buns and fries just stand in the way of the meat that I want. It was true.

Huge buns and the excess calories from fries, secret sauce and lots of cheese are often the biggest problems with burgers, but here are a few ways to make them less deadly to your diet.

Hand Pressed Success

I used to work in a restaurant kitchen, making burgers, fries, and more at Farrell's Ice Cream Parlor & Restaurant! Their burgers were really good, and because of their popularity, I hand pressed hundreds of patties a day.

The secret of a good hand pressed burger patties is to have something to press the patty into. When you use just your hands to form the patty, you end up with that weird shrunken patty that turns into an unsatisfying meatball in the skillet. Instead of using two hands to pat the patty into shape, use that burger press you got as a wedding present or even just a jar lid. I have a collection of various sized jar and canister lids that I keep in my kitchen drawer for just this purpose.

If you're making burgers for buns, choose a lid that's slightly larger than the bun, because they still do shrink when cooking. Lay the chosen lid down on the counter, drape a piece of plastic wrap or a produce bag over it, and firmly press the meat down into the lid. Use pressure to make it even and dense, and you will have less shrinkage in your burger. Use the edges of the plastic to pop your patty out of the lid, and you're onto the next one.

4 servings

Ingredients

1 ½ lbs ground beef (about 80% lean, preferred)

1 tsp olive oil or leftover bacon, sausage, or beef fat (unless using a non-stick pan)

Salt and pepper

4 slices of sharp cheddar (the stronger the cheese, the less you have to use)

Directions

Heat the oil in the pan or griddle over high heat until the oil begins to shimmer. If using a non-stick pan, you can skip this step and the oil. Cook the burgers until golden brown and slightly charred on the first side, about 3 minutes. Flip the burgers. Resist the urge to turn the burgers multiple times, though. Cook the burgers until nicely browned and slightly charred on the second side, 4 minutes for medium rare or until cooked to desired degree of doneness.

When you've got about a minute left, add cheese, if desired. Cover the pan or tent with foil if you want to melt the cheese further.

Serve on buns, or using the following suggestions to fancy up your burger and make it your own.

Chili size – This is an old fashioned diner dish, featuring a burger patty covered with chili. Use leftover chili or a healthy canned variety. If your calories and diet allow it, top with a little bit of shredded sharp cheddar.

Toppings – Two slices of bacon and maybe some cheese, the healthy fats of an avocado, smothered in mushrooms and topped with a slice of Swiss cheese.

Cheeseburger Salad – Make yourself a large green salad and then put the patty right on top. Instead of dressing, squirt mustard and ketchup on top, along with slices or tomato, pickles, and onions. If your calories allow it, a little secret sauce (aka diet Thousand Island dressing) shouldn't be out of the question.

Mahi Mahi with Roasted Red Pepper Sauce

This recipe is a little more complicated than some of the others, but it's certainly worth trying after you've gained a little cooking confidence.

Make the sauce first because the fish cooks quickly. You can also make the sauce ahead of time or in a double batch for other uses. It stores well in the refrigerator for a couple of days, and you can reheat it on the stove before serving.

Serves 4

Ingredients (Mahi Mahi)

4 Mahi Mahi fillets

¼ cup sesame seeds

1 tbsp light olive oil

½ tsp salt

Sesame seeds for garnishing

Ingredients (Roasted Red Pepper Sauce)

3 large red or yellow bell peppers or 3 canned or jarred roasted peppers

1 tsp olive oil

¼ cup chopped onion

2 cloves garlic, minced

4 fresh large basil leaves or ½ tsp dried basil

¼ tsp cayenne pepper

¼ tsp black pepper

1 cup chicken broth

½ cup cream

Salt to taste

Directions – Roasted Red Pepper Sauce

You need to make the sauce before you cook the fish, so start here.

If you don't want to roast your own peppers, you can buy jarred or canned peppers at most supermarkets and places like Trader Joe's, not to mention specialty markets that feature foods from the Mediterranean area. I love home roasted peppers, but sometimes it's just not worth the time and effort.

If you want to roast them yourself, then roast the whole peppers over an open flame on the stove, on the grill, or in the broiler. Keep turning them with tongs until the surface is charred and mostly black. Immediately seal in a plastic bowl or zipper bag for ten to twenty minutes. Take them out, one at a time, and submerge them in cold water, rubbing the skins off with your hands. A lot of blackened spots will remain, and that's okay. Cut open the peppers and remove seeds.

Whether you made your own roasted peppers or got them in a jar, coarsely chop them and add them to a medium sized saucepan. Put the heat on high, and add the oil, onion, garlic, basil, salt, cayenne pepper and black pepper to the roasted peppers. Cook for about 3-5 minutes. Add the broth to the pepper mixture and bring to a boil. Reduce heat and simmer, stirring occasionally, about 5 more minutes.

Remove the pan from the heat and pour the mixture into a blender jar. Let it stand for 5 minutes to cool just a bit, and then blend until smooth. Add the cream to the blender and blend for a few seconds to mix.

Return to the saucepan, and salt to taste. Keep the sauce warm, but do not allow it to boil again.

Directions – Mahi Mahi

If you haven't made the red pepper sauce yet, go do that first and then come back here.

Spread sesame seeds and half of the salt onto a plate. Lay fillets in the seeds, coating one side only.

Heat a nonstick skillet using high heat. Add olive oil and swirl. When oil begins to shimmer, add the seed coated fillets, sesame seed side down. Cook for 4 to 5 minutes on each side.

Pour ½ cup of warm sauce into rimmed plates or shallow flat bowls. Carefully, lay a filet onto the center of each plate, sesame seeds up. Sprinkle sauce and fillets with additional sesame seeds before serving.

Give the TV dinner another look

Eating alone tonight? In a bind? Don't feel like cooking and you're all out of leftovers? – Did you know that a frozen dinner is often a better choice than eating out, especially if it's fast food? Frozen dinners are a fixed size, portion controlled, easy to keep in the freezer, and not likely to be binged upon. Remember to read the label for the "bad guys," and keep the Healthy Diet Tenets in mind. Calories and satisfaction are key when choosing a frozen dinner.

Slow cooker pork (for soup, salads, or carnitas)

The slow cooker is a godsend for the busy family. It allows you to start the meat before work and have it ready to go when you get home.

8-16 Servings, so plenty of leftovers

Ingredients

2 ½ - 5 pound pork (pork loin, shoulder roast, country style strips, etc.)

1 onion, chopped

4-6 garlic gloves, minced, chopped, or pressed

1 tbsp cumin, ground

1 tbsp oregano, dried

6-8 bay leaves

1 tsp salt

1 grapefruit or large orange

Directions

Place the pork into the slow cooker, and add enough water to almost cover the meat. Add the onions, herbs, spices, and salt. Peel the fruit, then slice it into rounds and arrange on top of the pork. If you have extra fruit, put it into the water.

Cook on low all day or on high for 4-5 hours.

If you make a large amount, you can make multiple dishes with one batch of meat.

Pork Pot Roast – Right out of the slow cooker, this pork makes a delicious main dish when served alongside your vegetables or salads. Eat it just like you would a beef pot roast or pork roast.

Carnitas – Pull or shred the pork, then serve as is or broil it a bit to give it some crispy ends. Serve as taco meat (instructions under "tacos," below) and reserve the broth for other uses.

Pozole (aka pork and hominy soup) – See the recipe in the soup section for pozole instructions, using some of this slow cooker pork and broth instead of the pork strips and chicken broth in the soup recipe.

Slow cooker beef pot roast

Like our slow cooker pork, this is an easy way to make a "roast" for dinner and give you some leftovers for later in the week.

If your slow cooker is large enough, consider adding some or all of the optional vegetables for a great pot roast experience.

8-16 Servings, so plenty of leftovers

Ingredients

1 2-5 pound boneless chuck roast

1 tbsp olive oil, fat, or lard

1-2 onions, chopped

2-4 garlic gloves, chopped

2-4 stalks celery, cut into small pieces (optional)

1-2 tbsp rosemary leaves, dried

1-2 tsp thyme, dried

4-6 bay leaves

1 tsp salt

1-2 tsp ground pepper

½ cup red wine (optional)

6-8 large carrots, cut into large pieces (optional)

½ lbs fresh small button mushrooms, whole (optional)

1-2 cups dried mushrooms (optional) *

Directions

In a heavy skillet or frying pan, heat the oil or fat and brown the beef on all sides.

Spread the chopped onions and garlic (and celery, if using) on the bottom of the slow cooker, and then add the beef. Add enough water to almost cover the meat. Sprinkle the beef and water with the herbs, spices, and salt.

Cook on low all day or on high for 4-5 hours.

If you make a large amount, you can be setup for multiple meals with this one batch of meat.

* Costco has a huge container of dried mushrooms that would work perfectly here.

Slow Cooker Chili Colorado

This is a simple recipe, and can be as mild or as hot as you like. Many people don't realize that paprika is a chili, and it tends to be sweet and mild and readily available. I buy mine in a large pack at the local Persian market, where you get fresh and sweet paprika at the price of $4 for about a pound. If you like hotter dishes, feel free to use other ground, dried chilis. Just make sure not to use chili powder, which is usually a spice mixture, not just ground chilis. Beware!

Makes 4-6 servings

Ingredients

1.5 pounds beef (like chuck roast)

1 tsp fat or oil

1 medium onion

1 ounce dried and ground chili, such as paprika, California, New Mexico, ancho, etc.

1 tbsp cumin, ground

1 tsp salt

2-3 cups water

Directions

Cube the beef chuck or roast. Brown the meat in a heavy skillet, then place it in the slow cooker.

Add fat or oil to the skillet and brown the onions. Add the onions to the slow cooker.

Sprinkle the powdered chili, cumin, and salt over the meat. Stir to coat, then add the water and stir well. Cook on the low setting for the day, or several hours on the high setting. If you don't have a slow cooker, just simmer for a couple of hours in a heavy, covered pot over low heat until the meat is tender.

Salt to taste, and serve with grilled or roasted vegetables, such as zucchini, squash, peppers, and onions. If your family likes their starches, you can serve over rice, too.

Why use a slow cooker?

If you don't have a slow cooker, consider getting one. When you start the food in the morning, you come home to a house filled with heavenly scents of cooking food. Most of the work is done, too. Perfect for after a long day.

Slow cookers are available almost everywhere, so look at Target, Walmart, or your local department store. Until you have your slow cooker, almost any of these meals can be made on the stove top using a heavy covered pot, and a burner set to simmer. Most tough meats cook in 2 hours or so, so stick around to make sure that it doesn't bubble over or dry out.

Tacos

Tacos are a simple food, but visions of deep fried taco shells or the high calorie load of flour tortillas and heavy side dishes make them seem anything but healthy. But sit tight and I'll show you an easy and healthy way to make tacos that even my kids love.

Years ago, on a trip to Mexico, I ate a lot of street tacos (shocking, I know), and I noticed that they didn't fry the tortillas or do any of the fancy steaming that we do here in the States. Instead, they dipped them in water and then flipped them onto a very hot griddle or pan, turning them just once. When they were done, they were firm, but flexible, held together well with the fillings, and didn't have that weird taste and texture that comes from steaming, nor did they fall apart on the way to your mouth! Healthy, tasty, and practical!

Makes 10 tacos

Ingredients

10 corn tortillas

1½ lbs lean ground beef

1 jar of mild red salsa

Salt to taste

Toppings

Sharp cheddar cheese, sour cream, avocado, shredded lettuce, chopped tomatoes, chopped onions, salsa, hot sauce

Directions

Brown the meat and drain the fat. Stir in about half of the salsa and stir well. Salt to taste.

Heat one or more skillets over medium-high to high heat. Put some water in a bowl that's big enough for dipping a tortilla, and set it near the skillet(s). When the skillet is very hot, put on a wet tortilla and let it sit until it can be easily lifted with a spatula, about 30-60 seconds. Turn the tortilla and cook until side two can also easily be lifted with the spatula.

With a non-stick skillet, this doesn't always apply, and you'll have to test it for doneness by touch.

Repeat with the rest of the tortillas, overlapping them on a large plate, rather than making one tall stack (which can soften and steam them too much).

Serve the meat, tortillas, and toppings at the table, family style along with our Mexican Chopped Salad from the Salad and Vegetable section.

Note – Our Slow Cooker Pork makes excellent carnitas tacos if you don't feel like beef. Shred or chop the cooked or reheated pork and serve it in a bowl on the table. Green chili salsa (salsa verde) goes very well with carnitas, although you can never go wrong with red chili salsa.

Taco Salad

Taco salad can be made with the taco meat from the Taco recipe, the Slow Cooker Pork, a store bought rotisserie chicken, or virtually any other simple grilled or slow cooked meat, simply add salsa or one of the spice mixes that you can find in the grocery store spice section.

To make a salad more satisfying when you aren't having that big fried tortilla or refried beans, use chopped vegetables in addition to just lettuce. Lettuce is delicious, but it doesn't stick with you; adding cucumbers, peppers, and tomatoes can take a salad far.

Serves 4

Ingredients

4 servings of any taco meat (see Tacos and the introduction to this recipe for ideas)

6 cups lettuce, chopped

1 cucumber, peeled and cut into quarter circles

1 bell pepper, seeded and cut into bite size pieces

2-3 roma tomatoes, cut into bite size pieces

Toppings and optional items

Sharp cheddar cheese, sour cream, avocado, chopped tomatoes, chopped onions, salsa, hot sauce, tortilla chips, canned pinto beans (heated).

Directions

For this salad, I prefer to make four salads in four bowls rather than making one large salad. Distribute the lettuce and chopped vegetables across four large salad bowls and top with the meat. Allow each diner to top their salad with the toppings of their choice at the table.

The burrito bowl

The burrito bowl is all the stuff from inside the burrito, but without the outside (the huge tortilla). Remember that even though the tortilla is a big calorie bomb, replacing those calories with too much rice or beans can lead to a similar problem. Focus on the meats, salsas, and grilled veggies, with smaller amounts of cheese, guacamole or avocado, sour cream, and using just enough (if any) rice or beans to make your bowl satisfying to you.

This is another great opportunity to use leftover meats, by the way!

Serves 4

Ingredients

1.5 lbs of flank steak or skirt steak, trimmed of fat

2 tbsp paprika

1 tbsp oregano

1 tsp salt or garlic salt

Juice of 1 lime

1 tbsp white vinegar

2 tbsp olive oil, divided

1 medium white or brown onion, thinly sliced

1 green bell pepper, seeded and thinly sliced

1 colorful bell pepper, seeded and thinly sliced

2 medium zucchini or summer squash, sliced into strips

Toppings and optional items

Sharp cheddar cheese, sour cream, avocado, chopped tomatoes, chopped onions, salsa, hot sauce, canned pinto beans (heated).

Directions

Cut the steak, across the grain, into bite sized strips and place in a covered bowl or zipper bag along with the paprika, oregano, salt, lime juice, and vinegar. Allow it to marinate for at least one hour, but it is okay to let it sit in the refrigerator until you get home from work, too.

Heat a wok or skillet over high heat and add 1 tbsp of the olive oil. Add the onions and cook until they are the desired doneness and set aside in a large bowl. Add the bell peppers to the hot pan and cook until they are tender crisp. Add the summer squash and cook for several more minutes, so that they are slightly charred and tender. Add these vegetables to the onions.

Bring the pan back to high heat and add the remaining olive oil. Stir fry the steak until done.

Fill four bowls with the cooked vegetables and meat, and then top with any or all of the desired toppings, letting each family member do the same.

Serve with a green salad, if desired.

Personal Pizzas

My kids like to make their own little pizzas using just their toppings!

Premade pizza crusts like Boboli, English muffins, 100 calorie "thins" and even small pita breads can all make great crusts for individual pizzas. I've used small flour tortillas, too, but they are hard to pickup to eat. Your mileage may vary.

The key to having these as part of a fat loss diet is to find a way to keep calories low and the food satisfying. For most men, this means that the crust needs to be fairly small in relation to the toppings, while the toppings need to be healthy and satisfying.

It's often hard to get enough protein on such a small pizza, while keeping the pizza sizes manageable. We typically eat the extra meat on the side or toss it into the salad we tend to have on the side.

Speaking of salads, dieters should eat their pizza with a chopped salad, like our Chopped Vegetable Salad, topped with some olives, some of the meat that wouldn't fit on the pizza, and maybe a dash of strong Italian cheese for flavor, but be sure to make enough for everyone!

This recipe is per 2 Servings, but keep in mind that most men can eat a whole 8" Boboli, which illustrates the typical "problem" with pizza. As a result, this is a bigger meal than most, because it's hard to stop at ¾ of a pizza!

Ingredients

2 English muffins, 1 eight inch Boboli, 2 sandwich "thins" or 2 Pita breads

6-8 tbsp thick pasta sauce or Italian seasoned tomato sauce

2 oz grated mozzarella or other cheese

4 oz *precooked* lean meat like ham, turkey sausage, or turkey pepperoni

Toppings

Pineapple, onions, olives, etc.

Directions

Preheat oven to 450°

Use a fork to split the English muffins or "thins," but keep the pitas and Boboli whole.

Spread each with sauce, and top with cheese, then the other toppings. Bake for 8-10 minutes on ungreased cookie sheets until the cheese is bubbly and melted.

Allow to cool for a few minutes so that the molten cheese doesn't burn the roof of your mouth. Cut the pita and Boboli pizzas into slices. If desired, cut the muffin or "thin" pizzas into halves or quarters.

Serve with a chopped or green salad.

Salads & vegetables

Cheeseburger Salad

I mentioned this salad up in the burger section, but if you need it to be more clear, here you go! For the best burger experience, be sure to check out the burger pressing tips back there, too.

Serves 4

Ingredients

8 cups of greens

2-4 ripe tomatoes, sliced or chopped

1 small red onion, thinly sliced

Pickles

Yellow mustard (in squirt bottle)

Catsup (in squirt bottle)

Optional – secret sauce (aka diet Thousand Island dressing)

1-1½ lbs ground beef (don't go too lean for burgers)

4 oz cheddar cheese or high quality real American cheese

Salt and pepper to taste

Directions

Press the burgers into 4 or 8 patties. I'm partial to 8 slider sized patties, for what that's worth. Cook the patties to desired level of "done" and top with the cheese.

Chop, tear, or cut your salad greens into bite size pieces and arrange on four large plates. Distribute the tomatoes, onions, and pickles over the lettuce, and top with the warm burgers.

Drizzle the salads with mustard, catsup, and secret sauce and serve warm.

Chopped salad (Bulgarian)

On a recent trip to Bulgaria I was simply amazed at the sheer simplicity of their salads. Not only simple, but far healthier than the salads that we typically eat in America – raw veggies, chopped fresh and crisp, not a leaf of lettuce, and very little dressing. On paper, a lot of chopped veggies sounds like salsa, but that's not a fair comparison. This chopped salad, and the ones that follow, are fuller, crispier, and crunchier than salsa, and very satisfying on their own.

In America, we expect a salad to be lettuce based, but remember that we also have things like fruit salads, macaroni salads, egg salads, tuna salads… and don't make me bring up Ambrosia! Let go of the lettuce and try these out.

This is a great way to eat raw vegetables. Raw veggies take longer to eat than cooked, require plenty of chewing, and tend to be more satisfying and filling than the salads we are used to. Also, they don't require a heavy dressing, so calories are more easily managed!

Rumor has it that the Bulgarians invented the salad. All salads likely sprang from this one.

Serves 4

Ingredients

4 large or 6 medium tomatoes

4 Persian cucumbers (not peeled) or 1 large American cucumber (peeled)

1 large bell pepper (any color, but yellow or orange look cool)

¼ cup chopped parsley

Salt to taste

Onion (optional) – I like a little slivered red onion that's easy for others to pick out, but green onion is a milder alternative.

Olive oil and vinegar (optional) – the juice of the tomato tends to provide plenty of 'dressing" and you may find this unnecessary. Serve on the side if you like.

Directions

Chop the tomatoes into bite size pieces and transfer them, juice and all, to a large bowl.

If using typical American cucumbers (where the skin may be bitter), you may wish to peel them or partially peel them by removing strips of the skin with a vegetable peeler. English, Persian, and pickling cucumbers have thinner skins that you can usually leave on. Chop the cucumber into bite size pieces and add to the bowl.

Seed the pepper and chop into bite size pieces and add to the bowl.

Add the chopped parsley or cilantro, vinegar, and salt. If using onion, you can add that in now, as well.

Stir well and allow it to sit at room temperature for at least ten minutes. Longer is just fine, it's just vegetables.

Serve it in salad bowls because it's juicy, and have salt and olive oil on hand for those that want it.

Variations

Feta Cheese – 1 oz of feta cheese on each serving of salad makes the salad a "Shopska Salad."

Hard Boiled Egg and Feta – this is a called a "Village Salad" in Bulgaria. Sprinkle each salad with 1oz feta cheese and decorate with a hardboiled egg, peeled and cut into four wedges.

Ham and Feta – The "Shepherd Salad" is sprinkled with an ounce of feta cheese and 1-2 ounces of bite size ham pieces.

Leftovers –Adding cold sausage, ham, leftover meat, eggs, and even other cheeses is a good way to have a healthy lunch or dinner. It's simple, easy, satisfying, and filling.

Greek Salad

As I learned recently, a true Greek Salad rarely uses lettuce. Most Greek Salads in Greece and the surrounding countries are salads of chopped vegetables. That's not to say that they don't like or use lettuce, but they aren't as in love with lettuce as

Americans. This version does include *some* lettuce, but feel free to leave it out and call it more authentic.

Serves 4

Ingredients

4 cups romaine lettuce, roughly chopped into bite size pieces

4 large or 6 medium tomatoes, cut into bite size pieces

4 Persian cucumbers (not peeled) or 1 large American cucumber (peeled)

1 green bell pepper, seeded and cut into rings, then halved

1 red onion, peeled and cut into rings, then halved

1 tbsp dried oregano

1 tbsp vinegar

1 tbsp extra virgin olive oil

Salt to taste

¼ lb good Feta cheese, crumbled

12 Greek or Kalamata olives (pitted, chopped, or whole, as desired)

Pepperoncini rings (for garnish)

Directions

Use a large salad bowl and combine the lettuce, tomatoes, bell peppers, cucumbers, and onion.

Sprinkle the oregano over the salad, salt lightly, and drizzle with oil and vinegar. Toss lightly to coat. You can leave it in the large bowl or divide into four salad bowls.

Crumble the Feta cheese over the salad. Arrange the pepperoncini rings and olives over the salad and serve.

Mexican Chopped Salad

I'm expanding on the chopped salad theme, by veering off into the favorite cuisine of Southern California: Mexican!

This is almost pico de gallo in salad form. If it was me, I'd serve this with leftovers like pork roast or store bought rotisserie chicken that I picked up on the way home.

Serves 4

Ingredients

4 large or 6 medium tomatoes

1 large American cucumber (peeled or partially peeled) or 4 Persian cucumbers (not peeled)

1 large bell pepper (any color, but yellow or orange look pretty good in the salad)

1 small onion

1 tbsp chopped cilantro

1 hot chili (Pasilla is a medium hot, Anaheim is pretty mild, Jalapeño and Serrano go hotter still. Avoid the habanero; it's one of the hottest on the planet. Seriously)

1 tbsp lemon or lime juice

2-4 oz of a small Jicama (optional) – this is a crisp, slightly sweet vegetable that looks like a potato, but it's not. You can use jicama in place of cucumber if you like or use both for extra crunch and sweetness.

Salt to taste

Cotija cheese (optional) – this crumbly cheese adds a lot of flavor if you can find it.

Directions

Chop the tomatoes into bite size pieces and transfer them, juice and all, to a large bowl.

Seed the bell pepper, and chop into bite size pieces.

Chop the cucumber, peeled if desired, into bite size pieces and add them to the tomatoes.

Finely chop or mince the onion and cilantro, and add them to the salad.

Seed the chili and finely chop or mince, adding it to the salad bowl. Be careful not to touch your eyes or sensitive areas after handling the chilis. Ouch!

If using jicama, peel the skin off and cut it into small pieces and add it to the bowl, too.

Finally, add the juice, then salt and stir well. Allow it to sit at room temperature for at least ten minutes. Longer is just fine.

Serve it in bowls or rimmed plates (it's juicy) and have extra salt and the optional cotija cheese on hand for those that want it.

Asian Chopped Salad

Next up in the salad arena, the nebulous cuisine of "Asia." This is not anything traditional, but it is simple and tasty. It provides a jumping off point for your own Asian inspired salad, whether it's Chinese, Thai, or whatever.

Serves 4

Ingredients

2 large or 3 medium tomatoes, chopped into bite sized pieces

2 large cucumbers, peeled and chopped into bite sized pieces

1-2 green onions, finely chopped

1 large colorful bell pepper, seeded and chopped

1 tbsp cilantro, chopped

½ lb snow peas, strings removed if desired

2 tbsp rice vinegar or white vinegar

1 tbsp light olive oil or peanut oil

1 tbsp sesame oil

1 tbsp honey

Salt to taste

Bean sprouts (optional) – I love these, but some people just don't. They are very crunchy and can be unwieldy, so consider serving them on the side.

Peanuts or almonds (optional) – a few nuts adds a nice crunch and good flavor to the salad. Stir in or serve on the side.

Directions

Put all of the vegetables (tomatoes through cilantro) into a large salad bowl.

In a small bowl, stir together the vinegar, oils, honey, and salt. Stir well, and then drizzle the dressing over the vegetables. Stir to coat. Allow the salad to sit at room temperature for at least ten minutes.

When serving, if desired, garnish with bean sprouts and the nuts.

Sautéed summer squash

The accent over the first "e" makes all the difference. Without it, this would just be vegetables cooked in a pan.

Serves 4

Ingredients

4 small zucchini

4 small yellow summer squash or crookneck squash

1 red or yellow bell pepper

3 tsp light olive oil, divided

Salt and pepper to taste

2 Fresh basil leaves (optional)

Directions

Cut zucchini and summer squash into 2 inch long pieces. Slice each segment, lengthwise, into 8 to 10 strips. Seed the bell pepper and cut lengthwise into 2 inch strips.

Heat 1 teaspoon olive oil in a skillet over high heat. When the oil is very hot, add half of the squash to skillet. The squash should not be crowded in the pan or it will steam. At most, you should be able to see equal amounts of squash and skillet bottom.

Stir often, but allow the squash to brown in spots. Repeat with the second half of the squash, then with the bell pepper. Combine vegetables and salt and pepper to taste.

Serve squash on small salad plates or bowls, garnished with finely slivered basil leaf (if you only have dry basil, then just skip the basil, it's just not the same).

Grilled Veggies

Making good grilled vegetables is a piece of cake. I usually make extra to use in salad, wraps and soups. You can grill them straight on a grill or use a ribbed pan - the result will be the same - flavorful and smoky veggies in minutes.

Serves 4

Ingredients

2 yellow or green zucchini squash

2 sweet bell peppers

1 cup raw mushrooms

Bunch asparagus

2 large white onions

1 tbsp olive oil

Sea salt and pepper to taste

Directions

Cut the zucchini into long thick slices, the peppers in large squares, and the onions in thick rings. Halve the asparagus. Place all the vegetables in a bowl; toss them with the olive oil and spices. Once your grill is hot cook them on both sides and then serve as a side.

Option –You can also broil or roast them in the oven, or even sauté them in a large skillet.

Steamed broccoli with lemon pepper

You can use fresh or frozen broccoli to make this recipe, depending on what you have available.

Serves 4

Ingredients

2 lbs broccoli florets

1 tbsp butter

1 tbsp lemon pepper

Directions

Use a steamer basket to steam broccoli for 10-12 minutes. Remove from the pot, place in a bowl, cut up butter in small pieces and let it melt on top. Season with the lemon pepper and stir so all the broccoli seasons well.

Serve warm. If you want to serve cool, use olive oil in place of the butter. Feel free to top with slivered almonds and cranberries to add even more flavor.

Slow roasted mixed vegetables

This is a great recipe to make in winter, especially when you want some comfort food, but you can slow roast any time when you feel like flavorful and very satisfying veggies. The good news here is you can just leave them in the oven and not worry about them for hours.

Serves 4

Ingredients

2 - 3 sweet potatoes

2-3 sweet red peppers

2 large onions or leeks

2-3 medium red beets

5-6 thick carrots

1-2 tbsp olive oil

Sea salt and pepper to taste

Directions

Preheat the oven to 300 F. Peel and cut the sweet potatoes in thick fry pieces, bell peppers in large squares, onions in quarter pieces, beets in thick crescent pieces, carrots in thick sticks. Coat them with olive oil, sea salt and pepper to taste and place on a large cookie sheet. Cook for 90 minutes or until they have cooked thoroughly.

Starchy carbs

Starchy carbs can often be easily overeaten, but when made in reasonable amounts, they shouldn't be a problem. At the very least, your family may appreciate it, even if you decide to skip them tonight.

Easy rice pilaf

Rice pilaf is pretty easy to make, and it takes your standard white rice to the next level. Fancy.

Serves 4

Ingredients

1 ½ cups long grain white rice

1 small onion, finely chopped

1 tbsp olive oil

2 cups chicken or vegetable broth

¼ tsp ground pepper

¼ tsp salt

Directions

Heat the olive oil in a large non-stick skillet over medium high heat. Add the rice and onion, and stir frequently, until the rice is lightly browned and the onion is translucent. Stir in the broth, pepper, and salt. Cover and simmer on low heat for 20 minutes. Remove from heat and allow it to sit for at least 5 minutes before fluffing with a fork and serving.

Make it Mexican – Stir in some paprika and ground cumin just before adding the stock.

Make it colorful – For a little more color, how about some finely chopped colorful veggies? Carrot, green peas, or bell pepper? Maybe even all three.

Baked sweet potato fries

Serves 4

Ingredients

2 lbs of sweet potatoes or yams (about 2-3 large ones)

1 tbsp olive oil or coconut oil

1 tbsp salt

Directions

Preheat oven to 450 degrees. Get a large cookie sheet or several baking pans ready. For a really easy cleanup, line each pan with a piece of parchment paper (available at most grocery stores, near the plastic wrap).

Cut the sweet potatoes into slices, wedges, or circles. Try to get them to be similar sizes and shapes so they cook the same. In a large bowl, toss the potatoes with the oil, then sprinkle with salt, stirring periodically to coat them evenly. Spread them onto the pan in one layer. Bake for 15-20 minutes, then turn them using a spatula. Bake for another 10-15 minutes, until they are well browned.

Remove from the oven and allow them to cool for 5 minutes before serving.

Irresistible potatoes

Makes 2 potatoes per person

Ingredients

2 small white or yellow skinned potatoes per person

1 tsp chicken fat, olive oil, butter or ghee, per person

Salt to taste

Directions

Preheat oven to 450 degrees.

Peel the potatoes. If you have some sort of metal skewers, either actual potato nails or just some simple metal skewers for bbq or kebabs, skewer the potatoes, lengthwise. Using a sharp knife, slice down toward the skewer, slicing crosswise through the potato. Slice down until you hit the nail. Leave the nails in for faster cooking.

Place each potato, cut side up, in a shallow cooking pan or pie plates. Salt each potato and top each one with a dollop of fat or butter. When cooking, the fat will melt and pool in the pan, and a nice crust should form on the bottoms. Good stuff.

Place in the oven and cook for 30-45 minutes (longer times without the metal skewers). The potatoes are done when the slices can be easily separated when touched or when the bases can be pierced with a fork.

Remove the skewers before serving.

Charred Corn

Sweet, fresh corn on the cob can almost be eaten raw, it's that good. Still it's better hot, and especially good with some grilled meat. The only issue is boiling that huge pot of water out by the grill. Solution? Grill the corn, right alongside the meat.

Serves 4

Ingredients

4 ears of corn, husked and cleaned of strings

Butter (optional)

Salt to taste (optional)

Directions

Lightly char each ear of corn on a very hot grill (or even over the open flame of a gas burning stove). It will hiss, sputter, and pop. A lot. Let it.

When each ear is evenly charred and hot, serve.

If desired, brush with a little butter, and salt to taste, but fresh corn is so good that you probably don't need to.

Soup, stews, and casseroles

In countries other than the United States, people eat soup year round. No need to wait until it's cold and wintery, just have soup whenever you want. If someone questions you, just say "in countries other than the United States, they eat soup year round," then hand them a bowl.

What's with stew? Stew is thick soup, just like soup is thin stew. Sure, there are traditional differences, just like some soups are bisques and chowders, but they all come down to rules that aren't actually rules to begin with. Guidelines and rumors...

Chicken broth

Homemade chicken stock is far better than canned or boxed, and definitely better than instant!

For about the cost of a couple of cans of broth, you can make your own AND have chicken to eat, too. Bargain city!

Makes 3-4 quarts of broth

Ingredients

1 chicken

1 onion, halved (or a lot of onion scraps and peels)

1 bundle of parsley (optional)

3 bay leaves

10 peppercorns (or ground pepper)

1 tsp salt

3-4 quarts water

Directions

Remove the bag of giblets from the chicken and set them aside until you get down to the next recipe. Feel free to put them into the broth if you'd really eat them, but do you really want to find a heart on your spoon, nestled between a carrot and potato? You choose. But, be extra careful with the liver; it's gross and makes things taste like liver.

Put everything in a big pot and bring it to a simmer. Allow it to gently simmer for an hour and 30 minutes, but do not boil it.

Remove the chicken from the broth (yes, that liquid, formerly water, is now actual broth. True fact!) and set aside. Allow the chicken to cool until you can handle it comfortably, and then pull it from the bones. Chop it or shred it and use it for your soup or another dish.

At this point, you have chicken broth, so you can strain it, make soup or whatever with it, put it in jars, or freeze it in plastic storage containers.

Balkan meatball soup

This soup is the way you can have your meatballs and your soup all in one. It's one of our family's favorites, since we love ground beef and this is a really cool way to enjoy meatballs. It's also super quick - you can make it and just let it cook while you squeeze in a quick workout.

Serves 8

Ingredients for the meatballs

½ cup rice, dry

2 lbs lean ground meat (beef, turkey, pork, lamb, bison, etc.)

1 ½ tbsp ground cumin

2 tsp black pepper

3 tbsp sea salt

Ingredients for the soup

4 stalks celery

4 large carrots

2 zucchini squash

2 cups mushrooms

1 onion

Directions

Bring a large pot of water to a boil - ½ gallon is a good start to this soup. In the meantime, rinse and drain the rice. Mix the ground beef and the spices and add the rice. Form small meatballs, slightly smaller than a golf ball (think Swedish meatball size). Drop them in the boiling water. In about 5-6 minutes, some scum and fat will rise to the top. Use a spoon to remove it. Prepare the vegetables: wash and peel the carrots, cut them in thick circles, wash and chop the celery, wash and cut the zucchini in cubes, wash and keep mushrooms whole if they are small, or chop as you like them to be, peel and chop the onion. Add all veggies to the soup, cover, add water as necessary, salt a bit and cover. Cook for 30 extra minutes. Enjoy this soup with some chopped parsley, a dab of sour cream, or top with some green or red salsa right before serving.

This meatball soup is great the day after, so feel free to enjoy the leftovers for lunch.

Tip – if you leave the mushrooms out and serve with salsa, it's Mexican albondigas soup! Like magic, huh?

Tortilla Soup

Tortilla Soup is a favorite of mine. First, I love it, plain and simple – rich chicken broth, herbs and spices, lots of chicken and vegetables, plus the way we're going to make it, everyone gets to make it just the way they want it. It's not exactly buffet style, but about as close as you can come. You start with a basic bowl of chicken vegetable soup, and pass the toppings, taking as many or as few as you like.

By the way, did you know that, historically, tortilla soup was basically a soup of leftovers? Yep. Mexicans can be pretty serious about their tortillas. Corn tortillas don't have much fat in them to hold moisture, so a day or two after they are made, they aren't soft enough for a good taco, so soup it is. Leftover soup.

Because it's a soup of whatever you have in the fridge, keep in mind that no tortilla soup recipe is set in stone. If it sounds good to you, go ahead and switch things up.

Makes about 8 servings

Ingredients

1 tsp olive oil

1 onion, chopped

6 cloves garlic, peeled (broken is OK)

2 tbsp paprika

28 oz can stewed chopped or diced tomatoes

6 cups chicken stock (usually about a large can)

1-2 zucchini, or crookneck squash, summer squash, etc., quartered lengthwise & sliced

2 carrots, quartered lengthwise & sliced

2 bay leaves

1 tbsp cumin, ground

Salt to taste

2 cups frozen corn or 2 ears of corn (kernels cut from the cob)

1 deli cooked or rotisserie chicken

1 tbsp dried oregano

Garnishes (use some or all, it's up to you)

Tortilla chips or homemade fried tortilla strips (about 6 tortillas worth of fried strips)

Lime wedges

Shredded cabbage

Diced avocado

Cilantro, chopped

Salsa (red or green)

Hot sauce

Shredded jack, cheddar, or some fancy Mexican cheese

Crumbled cotija cheese

Cubes of cream cheese

Directions

Sauté onion and garlic over medium heat until soft. Add paprika. Cook until fragrant (1-3 minutes). Add tomatoes, broth, bay leaves, cumin, carrots, zucchini and squash (pretty much everything but the chicken and corn). Simmer for about 20-30 minutes, until vegetables are cooked, but carrots are not mushy.

While your soup is simmering, shred and cut the chicken into bite size pieces and prepare your chosen garnishes.

Add the corn and chicken to the soup during the last ten minutes of cooking. When the soup is heated through, rub the oregano briskly between your hands, crumbling it over the soup. Make sure everyone sees this part. You'll seem cool and mysterious, like you've been watching all the best cooking shows.

Top with desired garnishes and eat up.

Pozole (Mexican pork and hominy stew)

Makes about 8 servings

Ingredients

6 cups chicken stock

2 lbs country style pork strips, trimmed of fat

1 onion (white or yellow), peeled and cut into wedges

3 bay leaves

1 tbsp dried oregano

1 tbsp cumin seeds, ground

2 teaspoons salt

3 carrots, peeled if you like, and cut into disks

1 can (14-15 oz) yellow or white hominy, drained

1 cup fresh (or frozen) corn kernels

4 thin zucchini and/or yellow summer squash, cut into disks

1 red bell pepper, chopped into bite size pieces

Additional salt to taste

Garnishes

Green chili salsa

Cilantro

Lime wedges

Directions

Using a large pan or pot with a lid, brown all sides of the pork. Move the pork to a bowl and brown the onions in the pan. When the onions are almost done and lightly browned, stir in the oregano and cumin, cooking until fragrant (about 30 to 60 seconds).

Return the pork to the pot along with the onion, adding enough of the chicken stock from the pot to just cover the pork strips. Add the salt, and then cover the pan, slowly simmering the pork strips. Add stock or water periodically to keep the level of liquid adequate.

When the pork is tender enough to pull apart with two forks, remove it from the liquid and set aside to cool a bit.

Add sliced carrots and drained hominy to the pot and bring to a simmer once again. Simmer for half an hour.

While the carrots cook, pull the pork into bite size pieces.

When the carrots are tender enough, add the squash, bell pepper, corn kernels, and pork to the pot. Simmer for 10 to 15 minutes.

Serve with green chili salsa, cilantro, and lime wedges.

This seems like another leftover soup to me. Feel free to experiment. I do.

Tomato soup

Making a deep and rich tasting tomato soup in 5 minutes is a mission impossible, but you can do it our way and save tons of time without compromising flavor.

Makes 4 servings

Ingredients

4 cups canned tomatoes

4 sundried tomatoes

2 large onions

2 tbsp olive oil

2 bay leaves

Salt and pepper to taste

Directions

Clean, peel and chop the onion. Cook it in the olive oil over medium heat until it has developed a nice and sweet aroma. Add the bay leaf and stir. Once the onions are done, remove the bay leaves, transfer the onion to a blender, and puree them with the canned tomatoes and dried tomatoes. Season with the salt and pepper and return to the pot. Cook for an extra 2 minutes.

Tip – Enjoy this soup with some grated cheddar or grilled cheese tortillas. This is how to make them: Take a small tortilla and a hot skillet and cook it on one side. Flip over, sprinkle 1 oz cheddar cheese inside, fold and cook on both sides. The cheese melts deliciously, and makes this the best thing to dip in soup since the grilled cheese sandwich!

Curried cauliflower soup

I love the simplicity and flavor of this soup. It has a delicate creamy texture, with a slight curry bite, and a warm and comforting aftertaste.

This soup is even better the next day, so feel free to make it yesterday, so you can eat it today.

4 servings

Ingredients

1 large head cauliflower

1 large tart apple (like a Granny Smith)

1 clove garlic (optional, but highly recommended)

1 tbsp garam masala (aka curry powder)

1 tsp turmeric (optional, but makes for a nice color)

1 tsp apple cider vinegar

1 tbsp ghee or butter

Salt to taste

Directions

Discard the greens and leaves of the cauliflower, and then roughly chop the entire head, including the core. Peel, core, and chop the apple. Peel the clove of garlic, if using.

Place the apple, garlic, and cauliflower in a soup pot, with enough water to cover. Bring to a simmer and cook for about twenty minutes, until the cauliflower is tender. Blend with an immersion blender or in batches in a regular blender (just make sure to allow it to cool for a few minutes first).

Bring the soup to a slow simmer, and stir in the garam masala, turmeric, vinegar, salt, and butter or ghee. Allow the soup to simmer for a few minutes. If necessary, add enough water to bring the pot to eight cups of soup.

Makes four, 2 cup servings, assuming you added enough water.

Serve with a side of roast beef or roasted chicken breast strips for some needed protein!

Split Pea Soup

This might be the world's easiest soup.

6 servings

Ingredients

1 lb split peas, rinsed

8 cups water

3 cloves garlic, minced

2 bay leaves

1 tsp salt, to start

1 tsp pepper

Optional

1 lb ham (diced) or kielbasa (cut into circles)

2 carrots (optional), diced if using ham, circles if using kielbasa.

Directions

Combine everything except the ham and carrots in a big pot, simmering until the peas are falling apart when stirred (about an hour or two). I like it chunky, but you can puree the soup, if desired. An immersion blender (aka a "stick blender") works great here.

If using carrots, add them now. Simmer until they are the desired tenderness, usually another 20-30 minutes.

The meats that I've specified are precooked, so add them now and heat through, or you can serve them on the side and let diners stir it in themselves.

If it's too thick, simply stir in extra water.

Salt to taste.

Beef stew

If you have a slow cooker, stew is super easy, but the stove top will do just fine.

6-8 servings

Ingredients

1.5 – 2 lbs of stew meat or cubed beef roast

1 onion chopped

6-8 large carrots cut into bite sized pieces

4-6 stalks of celery, chopped

4-6 medium red skinned potatoes, quartered

6 cloves of garlic, minced, diced, or pressed

3-4 bay leaves

1 tbsp paprika

1 small can of tomato paste

Salt and black pepper to taste

2-4 oz red wine (optional)

Water

Directions

Put it all in the slow cooker along with just enough water to cover. Cook all day on low or 4-5 hours on high.

This stew will be very soupy, because thickening the stew is a very high calorie prospect. We typically skip that part and enjoy it, anyway. Salt to taste and serve.

Easy turkey vegetable chili

Makes 4 servings

Ingredients

1 lb lean ground turkey

1 tbsp paprika *

1 tbsp California chili *

1 tbsp new Mexico chili *

1 tbsp ground cumin

1 medium onion, chopped

4 cloves garlic, pressed

1 tsp olive oil

1 28 oz can of tomatoes, with juice

1 lb of misc. vegetables **

Salt to taste

* Depending on how hot you want the chili, adjust accordingly. Most paprika is not hot. California chili is mild to medium. New Mexico chili is medium to hot. Mix and match, as desired.

** These can be any vegetables, fresh or frozen. Tonight, I used a one pound bag of frozen green and yellow summer squash. No chopping! Other good alternatives are eggplant, fresh chilis, bell peppers, winter squash or pumpkin, etc.

Directions

Brown the turkey and drain it. Add the olive oil and onion. Sauté until the onion is soft and slightly browned.

Make a hole in the center and add garlic and ground cumin. Stir the garlic and cumin until fragrant (about a minute), then add the can of tomato and juice to the pot.

Add the paprika, chili powders, and any of the vegetables that need to simmer for a while (like winter squash or carrots).

Let the pot simmer for 30 minutes, then add any vegetables that are quick to cook (summer squash, peppers, etc.). Simmer for about 10 minutes or until the vegetables are cooked.

Salt to taste. Serve with hot sauce, cheese, and sour cream, if you like.

Sauces

Sauces are an easy way to take otherwise plain and simple foods to a new level. Simple broiled, grilled, or roasted meats become meals when topped with a sauce. Steamed or sautéed vegetables go from boring to delicious when tossed with a flavorful pesto.

Learn to make some of these simple sauces for those times when you don't have it in you to make something fancy and complicated.

Pesto

Pesto is a very flavorful paste that is often served as a pasta sauce, but it's even more amazing with roasted or grilled meat or vegetables. Try it on grilled summer squash, roasted potatoes, chicken breast, and even steak!

You may not be familiar with the type of pesto you're about to make, as most pesto in America is mixed with a ton of cream and poured over pasta. What a diet killer!

Traditionally, pesto is just a paste (pesto actually means "paste"), meant to lightly coat pasta, meat, or vegetables. Traditional pesto is much, much lighter and fresher tasting than the cream sauce versions, and it really lets the flavors work together. It does have a good amount of oil and cheese, so it's not super low calorie, but you only use a bit because the flavor is so strong.

Basil pesto is probably the one you are most familiar with, so we'll start with that one. Following the basil pesto, we'll give you ideas on other versions that are equally easy and delicious.

Traditionally, pesto is made with a mortar and pestle, but I suggest a food processor or blender.

Oh, be sure to make some extra (see the tip, below) so you can have it around to use with leftover meat and veggies.

Basil Pesto

Makes about 1 cup pesto

Ingredients

2 cups of firmly packed basil leaves

1/4 cup (1 oz) pine nuts

1/4 cup extra virgin olive oil

1/2 cup parmesan cheese, plus additional for garnishing

1 clove garlic

Salt to taste

Directions

Using a blender or food processor (much easier), blend basil leaves, garlic clove, 1/2 of the nuts, the 1/2 cup parmesan cheese, and the 1/4 cup olive oil until the mixture is smooth. Add additional oil in small amounts, if necessary to make a smooth paste. Salt if necessary.

Salt "to taste" is important. Parmesan can be pretty salty, so taste before salting.

Variations – Basil, good olive oil, parmesan, and pine nuts can all be a little expensive. Also, garlic can be very bad on the breath. Check out these variations to save money and cut down on the volume of mouthwash needed.

Roasted Garlic Pesto – Try roasted garlic instead of fresh garlic. You can use 3-4 roasted garlic cloves, instead of one fresh clove. Well roasted garlic doesn't really stink.

Cilantro Pesto – This one's my favorite, actually. Substitute cilantro for the basil and sunflower seed kernels or pepitas for the pine nuts. Cotija cheese makes a good substitute for parmesan.

Spinach Pesto – Spinach and walnuts is a great combination!

Herb or Greens Pesto – Almost any greens and/or herbs can be made into pesto, and you can use any crumbly cheese, any nuts or seeds, and virtually any oil. Play around. I love Italian parsley, and I once ran out of basil… it was really good.

Pesto Tips

To store leftovers, smooth the pesto into a tall narrow jar and float a layer of olive oil on the top to keep the air out. Even better, use an old ice cube tray and freeze it into manageable portions. Store the cubes in a baggy in the freezer. Thaw the cubes as needed, or even throw them whole into a pot of chicken soup for a great flavor boost.

Easy Mole

"Mole" is pronounced mo-lay. Mole is a rich sauce traditionally made with a million things. A million thing version of mole tastes great, but it contains a million things, so you'll never make it. Instead, I'm going to give you a simple version. Start easy, and learn to love mole, then when life is less complicated, we'll work on the complicated versions.

This version is easy because it starts with powdered chili. It's not the typical chili powder in the spice jars that people dump into pots of chili, though. That stuff is a mixture of spices, chili powder, salt, and anti-caking agents, and that stuff won't work. Powdered chili needs to be just powdered chili or dried powdered peppers. Think paprika and you're on the right track.

Powdered chili is available in many supermarkets, in the Hispanic food section, but a larger variety is available in Hispanic markets and online. Most people don't realize this, but paprika is actually just powdered chilis of a particular variety, so even the big bottle of paprika from Costco can do in a pinch. In Middle Eastern and Greek markets, you often find several varieties of paprika, from sweet to spicy. Reasonably priced, too.

Ingredients

½ cup of powdered chili and/or paprika

1 tbsp butter or lard (Yes, lard. It's healthy, remember?)

4 cups chicken broth

½ green tipped banana (this is just a regular banana, but still green at the tips)

2 corn tortillas or 1 serving of corn chips

1 clove garlic or some garlic powder

1 tsp cinnamon

¼ cup nuts and/or seed mixture (peanuts, almonds, mixed nuts, sunflower seeds, sesame seeds, etc.)

2 oz chocolate (unsweetened, baking chocolate preferred, but chocolate chips or Hershey's Kisses work, too)

Salt to taste

Water (to thin)

Cilantro (optional)

Directions

In a saucepan, melt the butter over medium heat. Stir in the chili powder until it's a paste, and then slowly stir in about a cup of the chicken broth while stirring with a spoon or whisk until combined.

Add the chili and broth mixture to a blender jar. Add the banana, garlic, tortillas, and nut mixture and blend until fairly smooth. It's okay if it's a little chunky, but if you can still identify a peanut, blend some more.

Return mixture to the saucepan, and bring to a simmer. Rinse the blender with the remaining chicken broth and add this to the pan, too.

Add in your chocolate and allow it to melt while stirring. After it's been melted and simmering for a few minutes, salt to taste. If it's too thick, you can add water to thin it out a bit.

Serve over chicken, turkey, or pork. If you like, garnish with chopped cilantro and serve with rice. Your family will like that, even if you're the only one not eating that calorie bomb!

Variations – An easy way to make your mole more authentic tasting is to use a variety of spices, different nuts and seeds, or a variety of tropical fruits and powdered chilis.

Great spices to try are cinnamon, nutmeg, cloves, allspice, cumin, coriander, oregano.

If you find multiple varieties of powdered chilis, use them in different ratios, depending on whether you like mild, medium, or hot.

Chicken Mole – When your mole is done, try browning a cut up chicken, boneless breasts, or a package of legs and thighs in a large skillet. Pour the mole over the chicken and simmer slowly until the chicken is done cooking (from 15-20 minutes for boneless breasts and 30-45 minutes for bone-in pieces).

Ripe over type

When using fresh tomatoes, remember that it's ripe over type. Tomatoes all taste different, but any ripe and flavorful tomato will be better than a bland and tasteless specialty tomato. Choose the ripest and the most flavorful available, even if it's cherry tomatoes.

Salsa Fresca (aka Pico de Gallo)

Technically speaking, salsa fresca and pico de gallo are two different types of salsa – both using fresh chopped tomatoes, onions, chilis, cilantro, salt, and lime juice, just in different ratios. Call it what you like, sound confident, and no one can say you are wrong.

It's very rare that a recipe requires a certain type of tomato. Even cherry tomatoes can be used in salsa if you like. Ripe over type. Roma, cherry, beefsteak, heirloom, red, yellow, orange, pretty, or even ugly. It doesn't matter, especially with salsa.

With chilis (aka peppers) smaller tends to be hotter, so in general 1-2 chilis will do the trick. Often, but not always, one large chili will give more flavor, even if there's less heat. Although tiny, one small chili might have your mouth burning until tomorrow. Taste the chilis before stirring them all in, just in case.

Makes 2 cups of salsa

Ingredients

1 lb of ripe tomatoes

1 medium onion

¼ - ½ cup chopped cilantro

1 lime

1-2 chilis

Salt to taste

Directions

This will be simple. Chop the tomato, onion, and cilantro and put them all into a large bowl. Squeeze the lime into the bowl, salt it a bit, and stir well. Allow the salsa to sit while you take care of the chili.

Chilis can be hot, obviously, so make sure to be careful here. If you have rubber gloves, you can use them, but at the very least make sure to wash your hands very well with soap and water after handing the chilis and before touching your eyes (and other sensitive body parts).

Cut chilies in half, lengthwise. The membrane is often the hottest part as it contains the oil, so scrape the seeds and membranes out with a spoon. Chop the chilis and add them to the salsa, stirring well.

Salt, again, to taste. Let the salsa sit at room temperature for 30 minutes to an hour, if possible. It gets juicier and tastier.

Garlic Lover's Chimichurri

Chimichurri can be a garlic lover's dream. This sauce is like the salsa or the catsup of Argentina, where it's common to find it on virtually every restaurant table.

I'm giving you two versions, one heavy on the garlic, which is more traditional, and the other a little spicy, but easier on the breath.

Makes about a cup

Ingredients

2 cups chopped parsley (not the curly garnish one!).

1 cup chopped cilantro

8 cloves garlic

2 tsp each, dried thyme and oregano

1 tbsp chopped, fresh rosemary (if using dried, use 2 tsp and make sure to let the chimi sit for at least an hour)

½ tsp sea salt or 1 tsp kosher salt

1 cup olive oil

1/2 cup red wine vinegar

Directions

Blend all the ingredients, leaving things a little chunky. Let the sauce sit at room temperature for at least an hour or overnight in the refrigerator.

Spicy Chimichurri

This version of chimichurri has less (and optional) garlic and a little bite of chili. It's absolutely not authentic to Argentina, but neither was the musical Evita and everyone loved that.

Makes about a cup

Ingredients

2 cups chopped cilantro

1 cup chopped parsley

1 seeded and chopped serrano chili

1 glove garlic (optional)

Juice of 1 lime

1 cup olive oil

½ tsp sea salt or 1 tsp kosher salt

Directions

Blend all the ingredients, leaving things chunky. Let it sit at room temperature for at least an hour or overnight in the refrigerator.

Be a Meal Survivor

You're hungry, busy, and late getting home from work. You didn't use the slow cooker this morning, and the thought of shopping, preparing, and cooking when you get home is more than you can take. Instead of flipping out, or worse, resorting to fast food, remember to check out Mealsurvivor.com before you head home.

Together with our friend Lisa Wolfe, of Miracle Fitness, Galya and I review only the best grab-and-go food choices from places like Trader Joe's, Target, and the supermarket, so you can shop for tomorrow and grab a quick and easy dinner for tonight. Subscribe to Mealsurvivor.com for regular updates, hints, and tips!

Lunch, to go!

Any food can be a lunch, and I highly recommend that you eat leftovers and simple foods for lunch, whether it's on a workday or a weekend; spend more time playing and less time cooking and everyone's going to be happier.

Leftover meat, chicken, turkey, meatballs and sausages can be made into sandwiches, salads, or just eaten plain. Some of my favorite lunches are simple leftovers like cold meatloaf, raw veggies, and some cheese.

If you don't have any leftovers handy, here ya go with some non-leftover lunches that are quick and easy to prepare.

Picnic foods & "leftovers"

Cold Chicken

Use "Roasted Chicken, Fast!" from the dinner section. Cut it up into servings and refrigerate them in zipper bags or plastic containers.

Hardboiled Eggs

See Smart Snacking's Hardboiled Eggs. Peel them and toss them into several small zipper bags, along with salt, if desired.

Meatballs

Meatballs are fast and easy, and handy to have around as leftovers. Make extra.

Makes 16 meatballs

Ingredients

1 lb ground beef, lamb, turkey, etc.

1 tbsp ground cumin

1 tbsp dry savory leaves

1 tsp salt

1 tsp ground black pepper

1 clove minced or pressed garlic (optional)

Water for simmering

Directions

Using your hands, knead and mix the spices into the meat. Form the meatballs into 16 round balls.

237

Heat a non-stick or cast iron skillet of medium high heat and add the meatballs, shaking and stirring until they are browned on all sides. Add the water up to about halfway up the meatballs. Stir every few minutes so that the meatballs are evenly cooked. Simmer until desired doneness.

Serve immediately or eat cold the next day.

One Bean Salad

This is just like Three Bean Salad, only less so. This is the essence of the bean. Just. One. Bean.

Serves 2 to 4 people

Ingredients

2 cans green beans

2 tbsp white or cider vinegar

Fresh ground pepper

Salt to taste

½ tsp sugar or artificial sweetener (optional)

Directions

Drain the green beans and put them in a bowl. Add vinegar, pepper, and sweetener (if using). It doesn't take much, if any, sweetener.

Taste the beans, and if they need salt still, add some.

Chill, if desired, then serve.

Three Bean Salad

This is three times the beans of our One Bean Salad, but still not hard. This is pretty classic American picnic food.

6 Servings

Ingredients

1 can green beans *

1 can yellow wax beans (aka yellow green beans) *

1 can garbanzo beans (aka, chickpeas) *

1 small red onion, peeled and finely chopped

1-2 red bell peppers, seeded and finely chopped

1 tbsp honey

2 tbsp extra olive oil

4 tbsp apple cider or red wine vinegar

Salt and pepper to taste

Directions

Drain and rinse the three cans of beans, placing them in a colander to drain.

In a large bowl, mix the honey, vinegar, and oil together with a whisk until well emulsified. Stir in the bell pepper and onion.

Add the beans to the bowl of dressing, gently stirring to coat well, then salt and pepper to taste. Adjust salt levels according to whether or not your beans were canned with salt.

* Green beans are essential to the Three Bean Salad, but yellow wax beans can be hard to find. Also, many people don't like the chickpea... other bean options are pink beans and kidney beans, but almost any three beans will work, as long as one is the green bean.

Just desserts

Earlier, one of the tips I gave you for cooking healthy meals that will please the family, was to change the game. By changing the rules, there are fewer expectations and less chance of a letdown. Just like a main course, the same can be said for desserts, instead of a really small bowl of ice cream or a tiny unsatisfying sliver of cheesecake, serve up something exotic, foreign, or fancy. Serve something they don't expect, you can always meet expectations when there are none.

Some of these desserts are more adult focused, like the poached pears and roasted plums, but if your kids will eat this kind of thing, double (or triple) them.

Poached Pears

Serves 4

Ingredients

4 cups red wine or pomegranate juice

4 firm, ripe pears (with stems, if possible)

6 tbsp mascarpone cheese

2 sticks cinnamon

4 slices fresh ginger

10 whole cloves

Pomegranate seeds for garnish

Directions

Pour the juice into a small pot, and bring to a simmer over medium heat. Add the cloves, ginger, and cinnamon.

Meanwhile, peel two pears and put them in the juice. Poach for 15 minutes, occasionally spooning juice over the pears. Carefully remove them with a spoon and place them in a bowl.

Simmer the juice until it has reduced down to about a thick syrup. When the juice is reduced, discard the spices and remove the syrup from the heat, allowing it to cool. It will thicken even more as it cools.

In a small cup or bowl, mix the mascarpone cheese with 2 tbsp of the reduced syrup and stir, making a thick cream.

Halve one of the pears, and scoop out the seeds with a small spoon, forming small wells for the mascarpone filling. Fill each well with cheese.

Pour the syrup over the bottom of a dessert plate, arranging the pears in the reduction. Garnish with fresh pomegranate seeds, and then enjoy.

Roasted Plums with Mascarpone Cheese

Serves 4

Ingredients

8 firm red plums or pluots

2 tbsp butter

4 tbsp mascarpone cheese

Directions

Put an oven proof skillet or baking dish in the oven, and heat to 400 degrees.

Cut the plums in half and remove the pits.

Add butter to the skillet. When the butter is melted, add the plum halves and stir to coat well. Arrange plums cut side down and return the pan to the oven for 25 minutes.

Serve the plums in four small bowls, each bowl garnished with one tablespoon on cheese.

Frozen Grapes

Frozen grapes are like candy, but they are grapes. Please don't eat all you can eat, but since they are frozen, it might slow you down.

Ingredients

Grapes

Directions

Wash and dry the grapes, then put them in a zipper bag in the freezer overnight. Eat frozen.

Fruit Gazpacho

This is like crunchy fruit salad, so if you don't mention the cucumbers or jicama, the kids might even eat it.

Serves 4

Ingredients

1 Valencia orange (or another juicy orange), peeled and chopped

2 cups pineapple (fresh or unsweetened in juice), chopped

2 cups jicama and/or cucumber, peeled and diced

2 mangos, peeled and diced

Juice of one lime

Optional

Hot sauce

Chili powder

1/4 cup crumbled cotija

Directions

In a large bowl, add all fruit and juice, stir well and allow to sit at room temperature for at least 15 minutes before serving. If it's a hot day, you can chill the fruit.

Serve the fruit gazpacho in tall highball, wine, or pilsner glasses. In Mexico, you'd top with a bit of chili powder, hot sauce, and cotija cheese. It's much better than it sounds...

Tip: if your kids won't eat this one, save it for tomorrow, when you'll toss it with some onion, cilantro, and sweet bell pepper. Serve over grilled chicken, fish, or pork chops. Instant salsa!

Caramelized apples & cheddar

Serves 4

Ingredients

4 medium Granny Smith apples

4 tsp butter

4 oz cheddar cheese (the sharper the better)

Directions

Cut the apples into wedges and remove the core. Slice the cheese into thin slices.

Heat a non-stick skillet over medium heat. Add the butter, melt it, and swirl to coat the pan. Add the apples to the pan and allow them to start browning, turning periodically to even them out. You might have to lightly flip and shake the pan to cook them evenly. Let the butter and the apples brown, but be careful not to burn it.

Place the hot apples in serving dishes or coffee cups. Lay the slices of cheese over the apples and serve.

Banana "Ice Cream"

Serves 4

Ingredients

4 bananas (previously sliced into rings and frozen in a zipper bag)

½ cup milk or coconut milk

Directions

Pour all ingredients in a food processor or blender and blend until it's creamy. If necessary, drizzle a tiny bit more milk to get to the desired consistency.

Other Banana "Ice Cream" options

Toasted Coconut "Ice Cream" – Before blending, heat a dry skillet over medium high heat. Add the coconut shreds and shake and stir until they are lightly toasted. Set in a bowl to cool.

Pina Colada "Ice Cream" – Toss in some pineapple chunks along with the coconut. You may have to hold back a bit of the coconut milk because of the pineapple juice.

You get the point, right? Strawberries, blueberries, peanut butter, nuts, raisins, etc. can all be used in various combinations. Experiment.

Sesame bananas

You can use bananas or plantains for this recipe. Plantains are less sweet and more firm. If using bananas, look for bananas that still have green on the tips.

Serves 4

Ingredients

4 bananas (green tipped, preferably)

4 inches vanilla bean (you can use 4-6 drops of vanilla extract instead)

8 small slices ginger

8 tbsp sesame seeds

2 tbsp butter

4 tbsp dark or spiced rum (optional)

Directions

Peel and slice the bananas in half lengthwise, then across into two to three inch pieces.

Melt the butter in a pan over medium to low heat, and add the vanilla bean (open and scrape insides into butter). Add the ginger slices and stir. Place the sliced banana on top (you can slice it any way you like) and cook on both sides. Add sesame seeds shortly before you remove from the pan.

Adding a tbsp of rum over each dish will make this a wonderful after dinner treat.

Tip: this also goes great with a breakfast of eggs and sausage. ...no rum unless it's the weekend, okay?

Girl Food

Sometimes you will want to make something that your girl really likes, even if it's less than manly...

Girls like simple foods that feel light and seem healthy. They almost want to pretend that their little foods are some sort of a "cleanse" so they'll feel pretty. ...and when they feel pretty, it's a good thing for you.

Note that most of these recipes are for just two people, so have a date night. If you think others would like them, too, just double the recipe.

Pumpkin hummus

This is the ultimate girl food appetizer. She will love it (and you!). Just remember to hold the garlic unless you specifically know she loves it! Sometimes Galya and I agree to both have garlic, or we both abstain - either way it's supposedly an aphrodisiac so might as well go for it.

Makes about 2 cups of hummus

Ingredients

1 cup chickpeas from a can

1 cup canned pumpkin (or baked or steamed yourself)

1 tbsp plain tahini (you can use almond butter too)

1 tbsp olive oil

1 clove garlic

Pinch salt

Pinch pepper

Pinch cinnamon

2 leaves of sage, fresh

Directions

Combine all ingredients, but for the olive oil, in a blender and mix well. Serve with the olive oil on top. Use vegetables, such as pepper, carrot and celery sticks for dipping. This recipe is super simple, yet it will make you and your girl go back for more.

Little sweets

She will find these sweet, thick, earthy and enchanting – these sweets will always remain a favorite treat for your girl.

Serves just 2

Ingredients

2 tbsp tahini or peanut butter

2 tbsp honey

4 tbsp desiccated (unsweetened, shredded) coconut

Pinch cardamom, ground

Pinch cinnamon

Sesame seeds and desiccated (unsweetened, shredded) coconut to coat

Directions

In a bowl, mix the honey, tahini and coconut with the spices, stirring them well with a sturdy fork. Form a ball from the mixture and let it sit in the fridge for 30 minutes. Use the mixture to make little candy sized balls and roll them in sesame or desiccated coconut. You will get 6 to 8 balls from the batch. You may want to store them in the fridge, especially in summer.

Almond Banana Protein Bars

This is a fast an easy way to make an equivalent of a fruit and nut bar at home. Girls love their bars such as Larabars and Pure bars. Now she can have a bar named after her!

Serves 4

Ingredients

1 small banana

4 oz almond meal and extra for dipping

2 oz whey powder

1 oz coconut flakes or fine oats

Directions

Mix all ingredients together. Form a bar shape large enough to make 4 bars after you cut it. Roll it in almond meal. Place it on parchment paper. Let it sit in the fridge for 3-4 hours, take out and cut in smaller bars. Coat the edges with almond meal and enjoy.

Walnut Olive Quinoa

It's no wonder that quinoa was known as the gold of the Incas. Because of its specific amino acid profile, it can keep you full for hours, you can have it sweet or salty, and it makes a good neutral base for the presentation of other stronger tastes.

You can serve this recipe as a salad on its own or just as a side dish; yet another way to enjoy the magic of quinoa.

Serves just 2

Ingredients

1 cup cooked quinoa

1.5 oz sliced olives

4 tbsp chopped chives

½ tsp sea salt

½ tbsp olive oil

1 oz chopped walnuts

Directions

In a bowl, mix the quinoa, cooked and cooled, with the walnuts, olives and chives. Sprinkle salt, add olive oil and mix gently with a fork to keep the texture fluffy and nice.

If you choose to serve the quinoa as a side dish, you can add some lime or lemon juice together with 1 tsp of lime or lemon zest.

Forest fresh polenta

You can make polenta from scratch or just buy it ready made.

For the guy in a hurry, I prefer to buy it ready - it comes in a tube, usually unseasoned, and you can serve it up any way you like, including "forest fresh."

Serves 2

Ingredients

4 one inch thick slices of polenta

1 cup mushrooms

¼ cup sprouts

1 ½ tbsp light olive oil, divided

2 tbsp sea salt

1 tsp black pepper

1 tbsp thyme

1 tsp turmeric

Directions

In a pan over medium heat, heat 1 tbsp oil, add the black pepper and the cut up mushrooms. Add 2 tbsp water or white wine and the thyme, and cook until all the liquid has evaporated. Set aside – this will be your topping.

Cut the polenta into 1 inch thick slices. Lightly dust polenta rounds with the turmeric. Heat up the remaining ½ tbsp. oil and cook them on both sides till they turn golden. Place on a plate, cover with the mushrooms and decorate with the fresh sprouts.

Tabbouleh

This Middle Eastern salad is our go to dish when we want something green and refreshing. Out with the lettuce, in with the parsley! This salad is unforgettable!

Serves 2

Ingredients

1 cup cooked quinoa or bulgur

1 big or two small bunches parsley

2 medium tomatoes

1 lemon - juice

1 tbsp ground cumin

1 tsp cinnamon

2 tbsp olive oil

Salt to taste

Directions

Cook bulgur or quinoa following directions on the package. If you do not have time, you can skip this ingredient and enjoy a more au naturel tabbouleh. Chop parsley finely. Chop tomatoes finely. Mix and season with the lemon juice, cumin, cinnamon, olive oil and salt. Mix well and let it sit for 30 minutes. Enjoy with pita bread, hummus or as a side to meat. Lovely!

Go forth and cook!

Taking control of your food at home is a big step toward getting and staying lean. I hope that you've seen how uncomplicated cooking can be from these simple recipes, but I also encourage you to check out the many 3, 4, and 5 ingredient cookbooks that are available in your bookstore.

Now, let's check out some next steps!

13

OK, now what?

You've come a long way since chapter one, and I hope that you've found new ideas and new hope for a slimmer and fitter future. It's not that hard if you just take things one step at a time, slowly and subtly modifying your life, your nutrition, and your exercise as you steadily change things for the better.

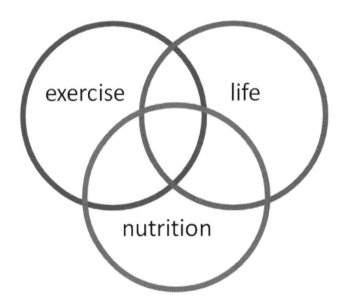

Before ten years ago, I'd lost weight many times, so what changed? Did I finally find that perfect diet? Nope. In fact, since I started on that last quest to lose weight, I've tried many diets.

What *did* change were my basic decision making processes and my resolve: I decided that I was going to lose weight. That is the most import point. Duh, right? But, of course it's not that simple. Like the smoker who's quit dozens of times, I'd always thought I'd decided to lose weight before, too.

This time, it was a stronger and deeper resolve, and with it, a plan that went far beyond "I'm going to lose weight" or "I'm going to lose weight on the _____ diet."

The plan was still fairly simple. I decided that I would lose weight even if the diet I was trying wasn't working for me. I decided to always look ahead, to see if there are other ways. Better ways? Different ways.

You have to decide not just to do it, but also decide that even if it doesn't go perfectly with your Plan A that you'll have a Plan B ready *before* you stop following your current plan. Never, ever go back to your old ways; have your Plan B ready to go. If or when you do drop Plan A for Plan B, you must start to develop a new Plan B, just in case.

A successful diet plan is not dependent on a specific diet. A diet is nothing more than a tool used *to* diet. It's not that different than building a house and having your crappy hammer break; buy another crappy hammer or a *better* hammer and get back at it!

So, you have the desire, the plans, and you've started. But by now you've done far more than just start. Depending on how fast you've read to this point, you may have done a few rounds of the Kickstart, made a few healthy dinners for the family, or even lost a few pounds by successfully picking some of that low hanging fruit and defusing a few calorie bombs. You started, you succeeded, you learned, and you have the desire to carry on.

This book is filled with specifics, from the need to pick your goals in chapter three to making specific, periodic changes using the training and nutrition steps in chapter seven. You learned what exercises to prioritize in chapter eight's Hierarchy of Fat Loss Exercise, and you probably learned way more than you *ever* wanted to know about calories and nutrition in chapters five and six.

Yes, there are very specific things that we can each do to lose fat and keep it off, but it's important to remember that we are all different people, with different bodies, metabolisms, jobs, and skills. While the specifics of how we each eat, move, and exercise will differ, at the most basic level, we all need to have a few common things in order to succeed.

As Galya and I learned as we interviewed successful clients, friends, family, and even other trainers and nutrition coaches, there are a few things that they all have in common (remember those 'common denominators' from earlier?).

Five common denominators of weight loss success

1. The time is always right
2. Have a plan
3. Have the next plan
4. Every meal counts & every meal stands alone
5. Permanent fat loss is the ultimate goal

These common denominators are important to reread often, so you they stay fresh in your mind.

The common denominators remind us how those who successfully lost their weight and kept it off did it. Learn from those who have gone before you, whether it's fat loss, business, or climbing Mt. Everest.

Knowing that others have succeeded and continue to succeed is important to build your own confidence in the process. Confidence that you can succeed is what it takes to keep moving toward your goal.

Next steps

Have I drilled the need to have a Plan B into your head yet? I think you got it, by now.

After you close this book, where will you look for more information? More importantly, where will you look for good information? As you know, the nightly news, magazines, and the internet are filled with good and bad info, and sorting it out is important. In Appendix 4 – Resources, you will find names of people, books, and web sites that we've found to be valuable, reliable, and accurate. These are the tools – you know very well that people can be tools – that I used to learn, and where I went to form my own Plan Bs. People like Lou Schuler, Adam Campbell, Alan Aragon, Dan John, Robb Wolf, John Berardi, and Mark Sisson are people who we've come to trust. They not only teach us the specifics of diet and exercise, but each also has a way to put things into perspective for people with normal lives. There's no "my way or the highway" with them, nor are their heads shaking with disdain when you aren't perfect. Reasonable people with reasonable expectations. No 100% compliance is required or desired.

"100% nutritional discipline is never required for optimal progress. The difference in results, between 90% adherence to your nutrition program and 100% adherence is negligible." – John Berardi, PhD

Social Support

Another important hallmark of weight loss success is having the social support to lose weight. Support can come from a variety of places, friends, family, or even a small group of like-minded people. Weight Watchers isn't successful because of its "points" or low fat diet, that's for sure! I know plenty of people who have struck out on their own, counting points and eating on the WW plan, all the while not getting *any* slimmer. No, Weight Watchers who are successful are so because of the social support of the meetings, weigh-ins, and get-togethers in addition to the system and diet plan.

I hope you live in a family that supports your efforts to get healthy and fit, but sometimes even that's not enough. Find all the support you need to succeed, whether it's amongst family and friends, a weight loss group at work, your softball or flag football team, or any group that you can rally to the cause.

From this book there are several example of social support. I actually met John Gesselberty and Kevin Larrabee online, on the JPFitness.com forums. We, and many others, found an online community there that's positive, supportive, and welcoming. JPFitness is now bigger and stronger than ever. You'll still find me there, too. Come on over, sign up, start on online training log, and say hi!

Spas belonged to Galya's gym, where members rallied behind each other and celebrated each success. Ryan was part of my early morning Nutrition Group, where I led a group of men over coffee, and we talked nutrition and training. Each week we shared successes and rallied behind each other.

I could go on, but my point is that a support group can be big or small, organized or casual, led by someone or just a peer group. You can find one to join or make your own. It can be online, like at JPFitness.com, or local held in your church, coffee house, or even your living room. The place doesn't matter. What matters is that it exists.

Get high tech

With the internet available just about everywhere, there are more tools than ever to support your weight loss goals.

• Join on online fitness group or forum. Make friends, learn more about fitness and nutrition, and even start an online training log.

• Start a Facebook page and ask friends and family to join

• Start a blog and share your goals, efforts, and successes

• Buy a Fitbit and tell others to buy them, too. Online, Fitbit friends can challenge each other and keep each other on their toes

• There are "fitness challenge" websites, like Fitocracy.com, popping up every day.

Learn from the best

Consider hiring someone. Some of us are great learning on our own, but others do better getting a boost from a pro. A good personal trainer can teach you new skills and exercises. Maybe you want to learn how to use those kettlebells you've heard so much about. Maybe you'd like to continue to train alone, but want a program customized just for you. Maybe you want someone to double check your diet, write you a specific meal plan, or help you lose those last five pounds before your reunion. These might cost a bit, but in the end you might progress far faster with the help of a professional than you would winging it on your own.

The skills of fat loss are fairly simple because they are built into us. They are instinctive, if we just surround ourselves with the foods, lifestyle choices, and activities that we were designed to have.

With your desire, your newfound fitness knowledge, and your new skills of fat loss and healthy living, you should have the confidence that you need to carry on.

Look around you, to the people who you know are lean for life; they don't struggle, because it's not that hard. This is normal life. Welcome back!

Appendix 1 – The healthy food trap

There are many foods out there that you may have heard are healthy. "Healthy" is a relative term when it comes to dieting. I think we can all agree that olive oil is healthy, but olive oil contains 140 calories per tablespoon. A few spoons of that stuff and you've taken in more calories than you would have with a couple of cookies. Sure, the cookies aren't healthy, but they may be fewer calories. Yes, it's an extreme example, since no one ponders a decision between a cookie and a spoonful of olive oil, but I hope you get the point.

Keep in mind the Healthy Diet Tenets that I told you about back in the nutrition chapter. Let's review them one more time!

The Healthy Diet Tenets

1. **Calories** – only as many as you need.

2. **Fats** – avoid the bad and look for the good.

3. **Vegetables** – fiber, nutrients... eat up!

4. **Protein** – muscle building and filling.

5. **Fruits** – it's what's for dessert.

6. **Activity** – either hunt and gather for the first 5 tenets or head outside to play.

Those are the six tenets that are important to your diet and health success, and pretty much everything you do or eat is covered in that list. But, there are things that tradition, hearsay, bad scientific analysis, or "the media" has done to leave us confused and misled.

The previously mentioned olive oil cookie conundrum was one thing, but let's look at a non-extreme example. We'll start with an easy one: natural peanut butter, or "Natty PB" in internet peanut butter purist geek speak. What does it contain? Peanuts and salt in its most simple form. In fact, you can also find unsalted natural peanut butter, which is just peanuts, I guess. Peanuts are healthy, right?

Yes, peanuts have good fats, protein, blah, blah, blah. So eat up? Not so fast. A serving is almost 200 calories, and a serving is just two tablespoons. That's not really a lot of peanut butter to begin with, and most people just grab a knife and spread, and if they measure, it's with a spoon, not an actual tablespoon. Even when you have the right tool, it's pretty easy to "measure" wrong and take in 250-300 calories when you think you measured 190. Oh, did you lick the spoon clean? That's another 25 calories, right there.

As you can see, peanut butter can be a pretty guilty culprit toward killing your diet, so look out. Peanut butter isn't the only healthy food that can easily be a diet destroyer. What about the peanuts that make up the peanut butter? Those are notoriously easy to overeat, as are almost any shelled nuts. Look out for those healthy sounding sports drinks (no better than soda…) and juices, not to mention the hippie-healthy yogurts and granolas!

To make things a little easier on you and help you weed through the dietary dogma, we've made up a list of some of the most common diet killers. Be on the lookout!

Diet Killers!

Low sugar, sugar free, low calorie, and low fat & fat free snacks like cookies and candy – The amount of fat is irrelevant to the calorie content of the food, and the fat is often replaced by sugars, and sugars and carbs are often replaced by sugar alcohols and artificial sweeteners. Read the label and don't let the low amount of fat sway you; calories are key.

Peanut butter (natural or not), nut or seed butter, power butter, or low fat or low sugar nut butter – Can be healthy in moderation, but keep in mind that they have 190-200 calories per one small serving! Weigh it or scrape the tablespoon flat to measure, and don't lick the spoon clean.

Nuts & Seeds – Healthy in moderation, but hard to moderate at 140 calories per quarter cup – If you're going to eat them, buy them in the shell and shell as you go. Portion your nuts out ahead of time.

Juice, "fruit snacks," and 100% fruit jelly or jam – It's not the same as fruit. It's pure fruit sugar, and sugar is sugar. They are typically not as filling as the real thing, so skip the juice, "fruit snacks," and jelly, it's just condensed fruit sugar.

Fruit – Healthy in moderation, but it can have a lot of calories. It's not filling to everyone, and just because it's natural doesn't make it okay to eat all the fruit you want. Don't do that. Choose fruits that are lower in calories and *satisfying to you.*

Whole grain breads, crackers, cookies, pasta, bagels, etc. – Whole grains might have more fiber, vitamins, and minerals than processed grains, but they still have about the same calories. Grain products add up in calories very quickly. Eat less of a version that you enjoy, rather than eat more of the "healthy" or whole grain version just because it's "healthier."

Food labeled "gluten free" – If a package of processed food is labeled "gluten free," it's still a processed food. Things like cookies and snacks, labeled as gluten free, are labeled as "GF" so that people who are intolerant to gluten will buy them, but they are still just cookies. The best gluten free foods are things like meat, vegetables, and fruit.

Diet booze, light beer, low carb beer – Lighter in calories, but the alcohol still affects you. If the buzz leads to more nachos, beware. Beer goggles make bad food look better too! Moderation is the key, so one *good* beer that you love may be better than three light beers that you only like.

"Diet" desserts – Diet desserts often lose satisfaction as they lose calories. Look at the calories of the dessert you're eating, not just a single serving. Would you rather have a sliver of a real dessert or a slab of some drab diet dessert? When possible, try to eat fruit and keep desserts to special occasions.

Cheese – I know people who can eat A LOT of cheese. Is that you? If you really like the taste of cheese, try sharper and stronger flavored cheeses, and use less. Fresh parmesan, sharp cheddar, and bleu cheese take less cheese to give you more taste.

Dressings – regular, light and/or low fat – To make up for less fat, low fat dressings are often filled with sugar or starch to give the dressing some body. These can add just as many calories as the fat you're replacing. – Choose dressings based on how much you're going to use. 1 tablespoon of dressing is not much, and if it's 150 calories, you could soon be in trouble.

Healthy toppings, such as guacamole & avocado, sour cream/light sour cream, cream cheese/light cream cheese or Neufchatel, nuts & seeds – Most of these items are full of healthy fats, but the high fat content makes them high in calories, but not necessarily unhealthy. Still, too many *healthy* calories are still too many calories. Don't be afraid of fat, but be wary of too many calories. Make room for these toppings if you want them. If necessary, cut other fats and/or calories (in cooking, dressings, etc.) to make room for the ones that you love.

Healthy fats, like olive oil, lard & bacon fat, butter, coconut oil – Yes, lard is healthy. Yes, butter is healthy. Yes, coconut oil is healthy. Still, too many healthy calories are still too many calories. Don't be afraid of fat, but be wary of overdosing on these things. Use the fats that taste best to you and use less of them. Stronger, more flavorful tastes mean less can still be satisfying.

Cooking sprays – The olive oil sprays are healthier than the corn and soybean oil sprays, but they still have some calories, despite the labels. Did you know that a serving of cooking spray is a .25 second spritz? – Can you count to a fourth of a second? Neither can I. Assume each quick spray is 5-10 calories and try to use just the amount you really need.

Turkey and chicken products, like ground turkey, turkey dogs, turkey burgers, chicken sausage, friend chicken, chicken patties, chicken with the skin on – The mere use of the word "turkey" or "chicken" can make a product seem lower calorie and lower fat, but through the magic of inexpensive dark meat, these products are often just as high in calories as the more traditional versions. If it's breaded or fried, it doesn't really matter if the meat underneath is healthy, does it? Breading = high calorie, so check the nutrition label and see how many calories you are really getting. Strangely, often the "real" product can have fewer calories than the turkey or chicken version, and if you like it better, you'll be more satisfied. Chicken fat and skin is healthy, but you need to be aware of the calories. Pull the skin off if you like, and calories go with it. Avoid breaded and fried foods and go for the grilled, roasted, baked varieties.

Meat, like pork, beef, lamb, bison, etc. – You know meat is healthy, right? It is. That old saturated fat thing is a myth, so I almost hate to point to animal fat as calorie bombs, but it can be (check out the calories and fat on a big ol' bratwurst!). Don't shy from the fat, but also feel free to look to leaner cuts to get fewer calories. Look for cuts labeled using words such as loin and round.

Fish, fish sticks, fish sandwiches, fish and chips – If it's breaded or fried, it doesn't really matter that the fish underneath is healthy; it's not anymore! Breading = high calorie foods. To be clear, please eat fish, but make sure to avoid breaded and fried fish. Sushi and sashimi are usually good choices. Ask for grilled, steamed, poached or baked fish at a restaurant, rather than fried or pan fried. When in doubt, ask your server.

Sports drinks – These drinks were designed to replenish carbs and electrolytes for high level athletes, whose performance is all that counts. Are you a high level athlete whose performance is all that counts, or do you want to lose weight? – Drink water and avoid sports drinks unless you are a true endurance athlete, and even then only use when necessary or when training for an event. Instead, drink coconut water or diet sports drinks that are 5-10 calories per serving, and in moderation.

Ice tea drinks, Snapple, Vitamin Water, flavored waters – These give the illusion of being healthy, but can be just as high calorie and full of sugar as soda. There are diet versions of some of these drinks, but read the label. Some diet versions still have 50-100 calories per bottle!

High protein snacks, bars, and soy treats – The amount of protein is irrelevant to the calorie content of the food. It's usually not a very high amount of protein and/or low quality protein, anyway – Read the label and don't let the amount of protein sway you.

Natural and "healthy" sweeteners like honey, agave nectar or syrup, brown rice syrup, concentrated fruit juice, Sugar in the Raw, turbinado sugar, molasses, brown sugar, etc. – Most sweeteners have a lot of calories, sugar or something more exotic and are just as unhealthy as white sugar. Don't let the claims of micronutrients fool you; if you are relying on your sweetener to get minerals or anti-oxidants, you're eating too much sweetener – Use a sweetener, the taste of which you enjoy, so you can use less of it. So, will you use less honey in tea than white sugar? If not, just use sugar. Will the distinctive taste of brown sugar allow you to use less of it in your oatmeal? If so, use that, instead.

Flavored yogurt, fruit on the bottom, whipped, and parfait yogurts – These are typically a little yogurt with a lot of sugary fruit that's basically just jam. Try plain yogurt and add your own fruit and/or sweeteners (if you must). Keep in mind that "light" and low carb yogurts are artificially sweetened, so they contain about half the calories of most flavored yogurts. Calories do count.

Fruit flavored cottage cheese – Cottage cheese with sugary jelly or pineapple stirred in... That's just jelly, you know? Try plain cottage cheese and add your own toppings. Also, try different brands of cottage cheese. Some mainstream brands are plain nasty, while others are very tasty.

Granola and "healthy" cereal – Again, healthy ingredients do not necessarily make a healthy product. Granolas are high in sugar, dried fruit, nuts, seeds, and often cooked in "bad guy" vegetable oils, then cooled and coved with honey or syrup. Calorie bombs, indeed. There are certainly healthier cereal choices, but keep in mind that many are filled with sugar and empty calories, and merely labeling them as "a source of whole grains" doesn't make them low calorie, satisfying, or healthy.

Have you noticed that many of the foods listed here are often advertised as "healthy," and use healthy sounding labels such as "fat free," "low fat," "low cholesterol," "full of anti-oxidants," and more? Don't trust what the advertisers want you to see. Instead, read the ingredient lists, the nutrition labels, and remember what you've learned here.

Appendix 2 – Popular diets

The good, the bad, and the fugly

Galya and I are often asked for recommendations and opinions on diets. In our opinions, a good diet is one that finds a way to limit calories, promotes satiety, and keeps things healthy, all without too much stress and effort. It has to be a diet that someone can live with.

In this section, I'm going to focus on the good (because it's the most positive and useful) and the really, really bad (because it's important and fun!). There are simply too many diets out there to highlight them all, so I am going to primarily keep to key concepts, rather than name names.

There are two basic types of diet; the diet that you believe will help you, and the diet that you believe in.

A diet that you *believe will help you* is one that you follow because you want to achieve a goal. When a little slip delays your fat loss goal, for instance, it might take quite an effort to get back on track.

A diet that you *believe in* tends to be easier, because you've bought into the idea that these foods are good for you. When you drift off path, you *want* to get back on.

It's a subtle difference, but the latter diet gives you internal strength (or a smug sense of satisfaction), while the former tends to elicit sighs and groans, and has dieters counting the days until the next "cheat day."

As you read through the following diets, consider how each might be more or less focused on fat loss or more focused on health. As you can see, the two are not mutually exclusive...

The good

These diets are *not* listed or ranked by level of awesomeness, but more by narrative flow.

Low Carb – Yes, meat and butter are delicious, but it's really hard to overeat them when you're eating them every day. Most of us have had the 16oz steak at the steakhouse and wished for "eating pants," but when it's your daily style of eating, you tend to tone it down. After a while, you can only eat so much meat and veggies, and the calories going in are fewer than you need to maintain your weight.

Also, by default, low carb diets minimize a lot of the "bad guys," which leaves dieters healthier and less inflamed, feeling better, and with better blood markers – such as cholesterol levels. Many doctors and health professionals believe that type 2 diabetics can succeed with this diet, maybe even coming out the other side non-diabetics. If I were a type 2, I'd sign up for this diet, rather than feel hungry on "everything in moderation" while counting calories and carbs.

The real trick of the low carb diet seems to be believing that it's good for you to live life this way. If you're on it to just get you there, all the while counting the days until it's over, it's not likely to work for long.

Paleo – A common misconception is that the Paleo diet is a low carb diet, but that's not true. Sure, Paleo has you avoiding grains and beans and focusing on protein, fat, and veggies, but if you decide to fill up on yams and taro roots, feel free. ...and last I checked, yams are carbs.

Another misconception is that you only eat what cavemen could have eaten. Again, not true, as a supply of wooly mammoth meat is scarce around most parts. Paleo dieters look at the *types* of foods that ancient man typically could have eaten and the types of foods that they couldn't have eaten. Armed with this historical menu, proponents looked at what these foods could do for our health by focusing on the good and minimizing the bad.

Sure, the caveman only lived an average of 30 years, but that's because they died from accidents, infections, and battles. Those who lived past the age of the active warrior or hunter tended to live long lives, relatively free of the diseases of today's elderly.

What's so good about a Paleo diet? It's a focus on whole foods rather than macros (fat, carbs, protein) and, as they put it, the focus is on "food quality." I'm not fond of that term, but the fact is that Paleos avoid foods that are likely to be allergenic, inflammatory, gut irritants, and thought to foster auto-immune conditions, gut, stomach, and bowel issues. As delicious as they are, bread, oatmeal, hummus, and other grain and legume foods are pretty optional in our diets, and the Paleo dieters tend to thrive without them.

Primal – Paleo plus dairy? This diet is the difference between a bunless burger and a bunless cheeseburger. You also get cream in your coffee...

Typical Primal followers focus on whole foods and limit dalliances into the realm of modern day foods rather than avoid them completely. An 80-90% compliance rate is often used as a guideline to get and stay healthy, fit, and slim. The line between paleo and primal can be a blur.

Primal brings to mind the noble primitive rather than the ancient caveman, so people who don't believe in evolution should feel pretty good about this, since there are primal people living healthy and happy around the world, even today!

Wise Traditions (Weston A Price) – Price was a dentist that studied primitive culture in search of dietary clues to dental health, but along the way, found that the diet plays a role in most types of health. Nutrition and Physical Degeneration, by Weston A. Price is the book he wrote on the subject. An oldie, but a goody.

This diet can be a lot of work, but they go a long way to follow many time honored traditions of preparing and eating foods like our ancestors from around the world did. Like I wrote earlier, our ancestors didn't live or eat perfectly, but most lived longer lives, relatively free of modern day diseases.

Unlike the paleo and primal crowds, the Wise Traditions people eat grains and legumes, although they take special care to make sure that they are high quality and prepared carefully. Grains and legumes are soaked, sprouted, or fermented to reduce toxins and anti-nutrients. In addition, there is an emphasis on raw dairy, fermented foods, and the organ meats that we don't often eat in this day and age.

Clean Eating – In chapter five, I wrote about "Clean Eating" in detail. In the fitness communities across the internet, Clean Eaters are making the attempt to eat the healthiest choices, and should be commended for that. People tend to make fun of them because they can get a little bit anal about their diet, but having been around dieters of all kinds, they do not have a monopoly on obsessive eating behavior... Not by a longshot.

There are Clean Eaters who live (and eat) by the rules, and there are others who "eat clean" and count calories and macros. A focus on health can give them the drive to carry on.

Real Food or Just Eat Real Food (JERF) – There are movements out there to avoid boxed, packaged, and processed food, which few would argue is a bad thing. Real Foodies focus on healthy raw ingredients, rather than calories and macros.

The only down side to using the phrase "real food" in conversation is that you potentially insult the person next to you by implying that they don't eat real food. That's no way to win them over...

The bad

This middle of the road category is filled with gimmicky diets that are hard to totally bash, but hard to recommend because they have so many questionable claims. Diets that stress the addition of supplements, require specific foods, such as something that only they make, require juicing, smoothies, or special shakes in order to lose weight tend to fall into this category. They probably won't hurt, but you might have to buy a fridge full of special meals or a $500 blender...

The "bad" section is also where I would put the USDA's food recommendations, which are still grain based, restricted of healthy meats and fats, and come with the advice to "enjoy your food, but eat less." A catchy, if meaningless, slogan if I ever heard one.

I will say that, despite the bad advice, if people actually did what the plan that the USDA suggested, it *could* work. But, it won't, because no one knows how much less to eat. They also suggest that people move more, of course. Gyms are filled with people who "eat less" while they "move more." This advice is not working, and hasn't for the last twenty to thirty years. The government's new and improved diet plan (at myplate.org) isn't really new, and certainly isn't improved. It is a bad plan, because it's not usable for most people, it does not provide methods to track progress and adjust foods, intake, or activity levels, nor does it provide motivation or methods to sustain it.

The fugly

These diets are dangerous or promote unhealthy practices. They might not make you sick or kill you, but these are the diets that tend to give you that "rebound weight" after you starve yourself and then make up for all those days of not eating by eating everything in sight.

HCG diets – HCG is a hormone that comes from the urine of a pregnant woman in the best case, a pregnant cow in the most likely case. Modern day HCG solutions are sometimes found to contain no actual HCG, anyway. When it is there, it's often so diluted that it simply can't matter.

What really causes the fat loss? 600 calories, baby! Why does it work better than other 600 calorie a day diets? It doesn't, as placebo controlled studies have shown. The reason you aren't as hungry on HCG and 600 calories? Because they told you that HCG will keep you from being so hungry.

This diet does nothing to teach you how to eat, so you are likely to eat all the weight back on again.

Low fat diets – These diets are misguided attempts at good health, and they work for a while, and then stop. When they stop working, it's usually because you are STARVING! Fat is a requirement for good hormones, and too long on low fat, and your body will cry for help in a way that you simply can't ignore – hunger.

A food that's naturally low fat is fine to eat, but foods that are made to be low fat are filled with extra sugar and artificial ingredients, leaving them often with more calories than their full fat counterparts. ...which were healthier to begin with.

Cabbage Soup – I don't remember cabbage soup being particular tasty on a regular diet, much less as the only thing you can eat.

Any diet that reduces calories will make you lose weight. A poorly designed diet, nutritionally speaking, will have you losing valuable muscle right alongside the fat. Cabbage soup is not a balanced diet.

Like the HCG diets, this diet does nothing to teach you how to eat, so you are likely to eat all the weight back on again.

"Cleanse" diets – Your body works 24/7 to clean your body. That's what your kidneys, lungs, skin, and liver are for, right?

A better way to cleanse is to eat pure foods (healthy protein, veggies, and fats), in the right amounts, take a vitamin if you need it, drink plenty of clean water, take your fish oil, get enough sun and sleep, and get plenty of exercise. Give your body the healthy nutrition and activity that it needs to do its job and your body will take care of itself.

Appendix 3 – Fats, oils, and smoke points

Below, you will find the full list of fats, oils, and their smoke points that I mentioned in Chapter Five. Keep in mind that smoke point isn't everything; oils can still be bad for you (soybean, for instance), even when they have higher smoke points. ...they just don't smoke as easily. Also, a lower smoke point doesn't make them bad to cook with, just don't go with high heat.

The chart starts with the highest smoke points, and goes down. For clarity, I have **bolded** some of the best choices for higher heat cooking.

This IS NOT a list of recommended fats, but an informational list about the smoke points of various oils and fats. If you look near the top of the list, you will see many expensive and exotic fats, with soybean and corn nestled right there among them (remember your "bad guys?"). I'm sure you can see why the world of deep frying and fast food has embraced these unhealthy oils (cheap oils with high smoke points = bigger profits at your expense).

Avocado oil – 520°F, 271°C

Safflower oil (refined) – 510°F, 266°C

Rice bran oil – 490°F, 254°C

Mustard oil – 489°F, 254°C

Clarified butter/Ghee – 485°F, 252°C

Tea seed oil – 485°F, 252°C

Canola oil (high oleic) – 475°F, 246°C

Olive oil (extra light) – 468°F, 242°C

Soybean oil (refined) – 460°F, 238°C

Palm oil – 455°F, 235°C

Coconut oil (refined) – 450°F, 232°C

Corn oil (refined) – 450°F, 232°C

Peanut oil (refined) – 450°F, 232°C

Sesame oil (semi-ref.) – 450°F, 232°C

Sunflower oil (semi-ref.) – 450°F, 232°C

Sunflower oil (refined) – 440°F, 227°C

Hazelnut oil – 430°F, 221°C

Almond oil – 420°F, 216°C

Cottonseed oil 420°F, 216°C

Grapeseed oil – 420°F, 216°C

Macadamia oil – 413°F, 210°C

Canola oil (refined) – 400°F, 204°C

Walnut oil (semi-ref.) – 400°F, 204°C

Castor oil (refined) – 392°F, 200°C

Olive oil (virgin) – 391°F, 199°C

Canola oil (exp. press) – 375°F, 190°C

Olive oil (extra virgin) – 375°F, 191°C

Lard – 370°F, 188°C

Vegetable shortening – 360°F, 182°C

Corn oil (unrefined) – 352°F, 178°C

Coconut oil (extra virgin) – 350°F, 177°C

Sesame oil (unrefined) – 350°F, 177°C

Soybean oil (semi-ref.) – 350°F, 177°C

Hemp oil – 330°F, 165°C

Peanut oil (unrefined) – 320°F, 160°C

Safflower oil (semi-ref.) – 320°F, 160°C

Soybean oil (unrefined) – 320°F, 160°C

Sunflower oil (high oleic, unrefined.) – 320°F, 160°C

Walnut oil (unrefined) – 320°F, 160°C

Butter – 250–300°F, 121–149°C

Flax seed oil (unrefined.) – 225°F, 107°C

Safflower oil (unrefined) – 225°F, 107°C

Sunflower oil (unrefined) – 225°F, 107°C

Fish oil – ? – maybe it's never been tested, because it's not listed on any charts. NEVER cook with fish oil, as it damages the fragile polyunsaturated fats.

As you can see by the butter vs. ghee comparison, it's often the purity of the fat that makes or breaks a smoke point. Extra Virgin is tasty, but the tastiness is in the particles of olive that are left in the oil. On the other hand, Extra Light Olive Oil is rather tasteless, but a better choice for cooking. Extra Light Olive Oil has a smoke point of 468°F, which is good, while Extra Virgin Olive Oil has a pretty low smoke point of 375°F. Both are healthy, but use one for cooking and one for places where you are looking for good taste, like dressings. There are some oils that should never be used for cooking, like flaxseed and fish oil (yuck).

Appendix 4 – Resources

In this section, you will find many of the resources that helped us to learn and teach about diet, nutrition, exercise, training, and motivation. Some are books, and some are the web sites and blogs of our friends and colleagues. Each is valuable in its own right, and I encourage you to visit them all and keep learning!

In addition, you will also find links to *our* web sites and to many of the forms that we referenced throughout the book.

Please note that the most up to date links are on our website, so if you just go to one place, TheFitInk.com/ManOnTop, you can find all of these links and more; just a few clicks, and hardly any typing!

Finding us online

The Fit Ink

TheFitInk.com – Galya and I write regularly on TheFitInk.com, which is our home base on the internet. To ask questions, make comments, and join in the discussion, our Facebook page is a great place to start: Facebook.com/TheFitInk

I love to get your emails, so please feel free to contact me at rdenzel@gmail.com, or either via our web site (TheFitInk.com) or Facebook page (Facebook.com/TheFitInk). You can also follow each of us on Facebook by subscribing:

Roland Denzel • Facebook.com/RolandDenzel

Galya Ivanova Denzel • Facebook.com/GalinaDenzel

The Fit Ink • TheFitInk.com & Facebook.com/TheFitInk

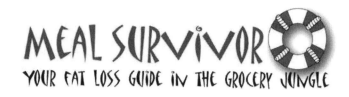

MealSurvivor.com – Created with our friend, Lisa Wolfe, MealSurvivor.com is an online resource for reviews of grab and go meals and snacks. It's only posted if it passes our taste and value tests AND meets our own high standards for quality ingredients. Meal Survivor keeps healthy eating within your grasp, even when you're short on time. ...and who isn't?

Downloadable Forms

I realize that books are amazing for reading, but they can be a little big to carry around during workouts, plus many people don't like to write in them. So, to help in this department, we have made many of the forms and charts available to you for downloading and printing at home. Visit **TheFitInk.com/ManOnTop** and you'll find the following downloadable forms and charts, plus anything new that's been recently added:

- Life Questionnaire
- Goal Chart
- Food and Activity Log
- Fitness Test
- Workout Logs
- Resource Listing (with clickable links)

Resources – supplements, equipment, and online resources

For the most up to date information on the resources, supplements, foods, and tools mentioned in this book, remember to visit **TheFitInk.com/ManOnTop**.

- Fish oil
- Coconut products
- Hard to find foods

- Foam rollers
- Dumbbells
- Chinup bars
- Swiss balls
- Books
- More

The reading room

New Rules of Lifting for Abs & **New Rules of Lifting for Life**, Lou Schuler and Alwyn Cosgrove – The whole series is great, but I recommend you start with either Life or Abs, as these two books changed the weight lifting paradigm, incorporating the most up to date info on core stability, mobility, strength, and health. We don't call it "the core" for nuthin!

Girth Control, Alan Aragon – Everything you wanted to know about nutrition, fat loss, muscle gain, and healthy eating.

Metabolism Advantage, John Berardi – A recipe for health and speedy metabolism in an easy to read and use format. John Berardi packs a lot of common sense into this book.

The TNT Diet, Adam Campbell and Jeff Volek – A tactical lower carb diet that can increase health and speed fat loss. It uses a varying level of carbs depending on your fat loss goals and progress, all without having to count calories, carbs, or grams.

The Primal Blueprint 21 Day Challenge, Mark Sisson – Look to our ancestors for simple ways to better health, strength, and sanity. Mark shows that getting primal in one's diet and lifestyle is an easy and satisfying way to get health and lean. A good book that takes you day by day toward the "primal lifestyle."

The Swing!: Lose the Fat and Get Fit, Tracy Reifkind – Training with the kettlebell doesn't get more efficient than this. Tracy distills kettlebell training down to the bare necessity; the kettlebell swing! The Swing! takes you through the very workouts that Tracy used to lose 120 pounds and to help her clients lose weight and get fit, today.

Men's Health Big Book of Exercises, Adam Campbell – For your next steps in training; this book brings you the big names in fitness. You can "taste test" programs by the best in the business. I'm recommending the hardcopy book, in this case. This book has many pictures of proper exercise form, but they are not formatted for the kindle.

Infinite Intensity, Ross Enamait – Do you want to perfect the home based workout? Ross Enamait uses bodyweight exercises and simple, often homemade tools for the ultimate home gym, all without spending much money or taking up your valuable space.

Never Let Go, Dan John – More a book of inspiration and fitness wisdom, peppered with golden training tips, Dan brings his common sense in an easy to read and entertaining book that's sure to motivate you for a long time.

Hearty Soups, Georgeanne Brennan –It's not a diet or health cookbook, but turns out it's *naturally* healthy. Very few ingredients, quick, easy, and delicious.

Art of Manliness Man Cookbook – A free, and manly, cookbook, just for signing up for their newsletter! Subscribe at ArtOfManliness.com

Of course, there's really no end to great fitness, nutrition, and cookbooks, but these are a great place to start.

For a complete list of our current reading recommendations, along with links directly to the books, go to TheFitInk.com/ReadingRoom.

Appendix 5 – The ridiculously detailed Table of Contents

When we produced this book for Kindle, we gave the reader the ability to "jump" to any point in the book via this section. Unfortunately, paper doesn't work that way, but at least you can find what you're looking for pretty easily with this ridiculously detailed Table of Contents.

The *ridiculously* detailed table of contents

Made in the USA
San Bernardino, CA
11 December 2014